Alpers and Mancall's

# Essentials of the Neurologic Examination

edition 2

Alpers and Mancall's

# Essentials of the Neurologic Examination

edition 2

Elliott L. Mancall, M.D.

Professor of Neurology
Hahnemann Medical College
Philadelphia, Pennsylvania

F. A. DAVIS COMPANY · Philadelphia

Printed in the United States of America

**Library of Congress Cataloging in Publication Data**

Alpers, Bernard Jacob, 1900–
Alpers and Mancall's Essentials of the neurologic examination.

Previously published as: Essentials of the neurological examination.
Includes bibliographies and index.
1. Neurologic examination. I. Mancall, Elliott L., 1927– . II. Title.
III. Title: Essentials of the neurologic examination.
RC348.A42 1981 616.8′0475 81-919
ISBN 0-8036-5805-2 AACR2

**To J.C.M.**

# PREFACE

This text discusses the neurologic examination, describes the interpretation of abnormal neurologic signs, and gives an overview of the more commonly employed ancillary laboratory techniques utilized in the patient with neurologic disease. It is anticipated that the physician will have been taught at least the rudiments of a neurologic survey in the course of training. Further experience can provide increasing familiarity with the methodology of the examination, an understanding of the appropriate, rational approach to the patient with neurologic disease, and a deeper grasp of the nature of the neurologic problem. It must be assumed that for want of time the physician may in some instances be forced to carry out an admittedly incomplete examination directed toward the chief or presenting problem alone. The aim of this text is to assist in the development of clinical skills in the performance of both selective and complete examinations.

This book is concerned with essentials and will aid the physician in determining (1) whether a neurologic problem is present, (2) its location, (3) its pathogenesis, and (4) how it should be pursued.

Among the many who assisted in the development of this new edition, Dr. Charles Brill was particularly helpful in matters related to child neurology, and Dr. Louis Pearlstein was of vital assistance in the preparation of new illustrations. Without Mrs. Katherine Breslin's unflagging enthusiasm and forbearance, completion of the manuscript would have remained uncertain.

Elliott L. Mancall, M.D.

# CONTENTS

# 1

# EXAMINATION OF THE NERVOUS SYSTEM

An adequate examination of the nervous system is essential for even an elementary understanding of neurologic disease. Unfortunately, such an examination is almost universally neglected among practitioners of medicine and is approached only with the greatest of trepidation even by students. A tap of the patellar tendons, a hasty appraisal of the response of the pupils to light, and a cursory evaluation of the hand grips all too often are deemed sufficient for most purposes. A proper neurologic examination is admittedly a complex matter, but it is unfortunate that it should be regarded by most physicians as hopelessly beyond their reach and too obscure to be attempted except by the initiated. Such shrinking from an appropriate examination all too often results in failure to recognize neurologic disease, particularly if it is not far advanced. It is therefore of the highest importance to indicate to those who are not themselves neurologists how to examine the nervous system and how to utilize the data so collected in a meaningful fashion. This chapter will be devoted to a description of the clinical examination of the nervous system itself; subsequent chapters are devoted to an account of the meaning and significance of the observations derived therefrom.

It should be emphasized at the outset that in a general way both the history and the examination are directed toward determining first, *where* the lesion is, and second, *what* it is. If this approach is adhered to, many pitfalls in diagnosis will be avoided. A proper examination of the nervous system itself is a highly systematic affair, and requires investigation of the mental state, cranial nerves, motor and reflex systems, cerebellar apparatus, and of a variety of sensory modalities. For special purposes, investigations may be made of the autonomic nervous system as well. It is on the basis of such a clinical approach that a rational differential diagnosis can be entertained, appropriate laboratory studies pursued, and suitable therapy instituted.

## THE HISTORY

No examination can be complete without a history, and no history can be too complete. The diagnosis of disease involves the careful collection and sifting of data, with the taking of a history as the first logical step. The importance of the history itself is underlined by the fact that an accurate diagnosis in the great majority of cases of neurologic disease is achieved primarily on the basis of historical data.

The recording of the history may follow two general lines: the patient may recite his story without guidance or help from the physician, or he may be guided by leading questions. A proper history combines both approaches. It is sensible to let the patient recite his own story and to follow this with specific inquiries concerning pertinent points of information that may have been omitted or require clarification. Any medical history is always better the greater the experience of the physician, a feature particularly true in instances of neurologic disease. The greater the orientation in things neurologic, the more pertinent and thorough will be the history. Despite this, much can be learned by aggressive curiosity and by adherence to the guiding principles that no history must be taken at proffered value and no symptom left unanalyzed.

All patients approach the physician with some degree of fear; hence their offer of historical evidence will vary in accord with their own personality makeup. Some will make light of symptoms and offer little information; others will make too much of symptoms and offer confusing evidence; yet others will attempt to define their symptoms in diagnostic terms and by interpretations of their own. The rare patient will present his evidence logically and carefully. Because of the patient's anxiety concerning his illness, his ability to recite his symptoms in a concise and sequential manner is commonly impaired. Insistence of the physician in separating wheat from chaff is essential.

### The Family History

The family history assumes considerable importance under a variety of circumstances. It is, for example, of major significance in identification of the spinocerebellar degenerations, certain forms of motor system disease, many myopathies, some cases of peripheral neuropathy, a host of neuronal storage diseases, the leukodystrophies, and many degenerative processes such as Huntington's disease. Migraine is typically a familial disorder, as are many instances of mental retardation, particularly those based on metabolic deficiencies. A familial pattern may even be found in occasional cases of multiple sclerosis or brain tumor, and the occurrence of seizures in other members of a family becomes extremely important in the diagnosis of idiopathic epilepsy. All too often an inadequate or missing family history may preclude accurate diagnosis in an individual patient.

When a positive family history is obtained, an attempt should be made to delineate as precisely as possible the mode of inheritance, for purposes not only of accurate diagnosis but of family (genetic) counselling as well. Care must of course be taken to separate instances of shared environmental exposure from true genetic derangements in situations of disease occurring in several members of a given family.

## The Developmental History

This is vitally important in all cases of disease of the nervous system that occur in infancy, childhood, and adolescence. Poor health in the mother may result in prematurity or in the appearance of one of a variety of congenital malformations. Evidence of avitaminosis, infection (especially rubella), persistent vomiting, hypertension, or bleeding during pregnancy must be sought. The question of Rh compatibility must be raised. Factors as diverse as maternal myasthenia, drug use or abuse, and alcoholism are of major concern as well.

Particular attention should be directed toward ascertaining whether the child was premature or born at term. Exact details as to prematurity are essential. The duration and nature of the delivery should be investigated. Prolonged or precipitate delivery, natural or forceps birth, and the mode of presentation are all important factors to be pursued. The type of premedication and of anesthesia and its duration should be investigated. The weight of the infant at birth and the condition on delivery are of potential significance, and particular inquiry should be made concerning cyanosis, jaundice, convulsions, and apnea. If initiation of breathing was difficult, it is essential to know the duration of the period of apnea and whether intubation or the use of a respirator was necessary. It is likewise important to know whether the infant was breast-fed or bottle-fed and whether sucking was impaired. Further developmental details concern the rapidity of weight gain; the appearance of dentition; the age of development of sitting, standing, creeping, and head control; the onset of talking; the acquisition of toilet habits; the development of skilled acts; and, in older children, the school record, behavioral patterns, immunizations, and occurrence of childhood diseases. Comparison of the patient's development with that of siblings is often of great value. No developmental inquiry is complete without inquiry into personality structure and development and quality of the home environment.*

## Onset of the Disease

An analysis of the method of development of the illness often gives vital information concerning its nature (Fig. 1-1). An abrupt or apoplectic onset of symptoms is found typically in cerebral hemorrhage and embolism; in some forms of brain tumor; in meningitis, particularly in the fulminating meningococcal form; in head injury; and in some viral encephalitides, to choose random examples. The time of onset of symptoms may be of equal importance, as in the early morning occurrence of cerebral thrombosis. The mere reporting of such an onset, however, is not sufficient. It is important to know whether the onset was with fever, pain, injury, convulsions, or loss of consciousness. Thus, acutely evolving paralysis of the legs with pain is something quite different from that without pain; in the former instance the orientation may be toward neuropathy or cauda equina tumor, in the latter, toward poliomyelitis or perhaps a parasagittal meningioma. Again, the occurrence of headache with fever suggests systemic disease, meningitis, or meningoencephalitis; without fever, disorders such as tumor or subarachnoid hemorrhage present themselves. By careful analysis of such details it may be possible to obtain important clues to diagnosis. It may also become evident that while the onset of the immediate

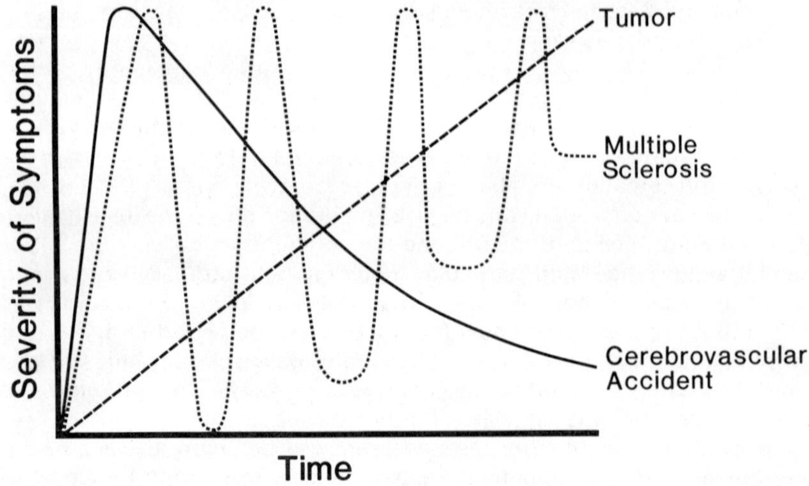


**FIGURE 1-1.** Contrasting modes of evolution in typical neurologic disorders.

*The Denver Developmental Screening Test of Dr. William K. Frankenburg, University of Colorado Medical Center, is useful for assessing the developmental level of children 1 month to 6 years of age.

symptoms was abrupt, minor signs of abnormality may actually have been present for some time. This is apparent, for example, in the history of transient ischemic attacks preceding cerebral thrombosis. Disregarded headaches may have preceded the seemingly acute onset of symptoms in instances of brain tumor, and pains in the back or legs, otherwise ignored, may antedate the sudden development of paraplegia in cases of spinal cord tumor.

In other patients, the onset of the illness may be slow and the development gradual. In such cases, one must determine whether the evolution has been steadily progressive or whether it has been broken by periods of complete or incomplete remission of symptoms. A slowly evolving disorder may extend over a period of months or years, and its beginnings may be so indefinite as to be lost in the past. Symptoms such as minor memory disturbance, increased irritability, or mild personality alterations may be so slight at first as to be disregarded, their true nature and significance becoming apparent only when the disease has become well advanced.

## Progression of the Disease

A determination of the nature of progression and evolution of disease is also essential. Progression implies continued activity regardless of cause. It is vital to know whether such progression has been maintained steadily; whether there have been plateaus with stabilization of symptoms for varying periods, followed by more progression; or whether there have been remissions, more or less complete, for longer or shorter periods. Whether progression of symptoms has been rapid or slow must be determined.

In Alzheimer's disease, for example, symptoms as a rule develop gradually and progress slowly but inexorably. The same is true for most degenerative diseases, for some infections such as general paresis or Jakob-Creutzfeldt disease, and in the majority of cases of brain tumor. On the other hand, paralysis agitans (Parkinson's disease) may develop slowly and evolve gradually, but with interspersed periods of stability. A more rapidly unrelenting course is observed in disorders such as amyotrophic lateral sclerosis and in malignant brain tumors, and a fulminating course may be encountered in viral or bacterial infections and in some metabolic disorders. A stuttering course with numerous clinical plateaus is often found in thrombo-occlusive disease involving large vessels such as the carotid or basilar arteries.

In some circumstances, recognition of a pattern of exacerbation and remissions is of the greatest importance in achieving the correct diagnosis. When clinical remissions are noted, it should be established whether they have been complete or incomplete, and, if complete, their duration should be noted. The outstanding example of a remitting and relapsing course is that of multiple sclerosis, but remissions may occur in other diseases, such as myasthenia gravis and even in some cases of brain tumor. Recurrent symptoms with varying degrees of resolution are common in cerebrovascular disease, and other disorders such as epilepsy, migraine, Meniere's disease, or periodic paralysis exhibit a characteristically episodic or periodic quality.

## Nature of the Symptoms

Once the mode of onset and progression of the illness have been determined, analysis of the main complaints follows. Careful appraisal of the various symptoms of which the patient complains is essential to an accurate diagnosis. However, one must accept the patient's own words for his or her symptoms at face value only with caution. Patients frequently complain of numbness of the limb when they mean weakness, or may complain of dizziness without meaning vertigo in the true sense of the word. Each symptom thus requires precise exploration. Examples of some of the more common complaints encountered in patients with neurologic disorders follow.

## Pain

A complaint of pain must be analyzed carefully, both qualitatively and quantitatively. Pain in any part of the body should be defined along the following lines: (1) the nature of the pain with reference to both its quality and intensity. It is often difficult for patients to describe pain accurately in this regard, but patience will often elicit helpful information. It is useful, for example, to know whether the pain is deep or superficial; aching, boring, burning, or throbbing; or lancinating and radiating from one part to another or appearing simultaneously in all parts of a limb; (2) the exact location of the pain, and the path of radiation, that is, whether it appears along the expected distribution of a peripheral nerve or spinal root, or neither, as is the case in central pain due to lesions of the thalamus or spinothalamic tract; (3) the duration and constancy of pain; (4) identifiable factors that aggravate the pain, such as movement, posture, climate, straining, sneezing, coughing; (5) those factors that relieve the pain, for example, whether relieved by drugs and, if so, in what dosage, or whether relieved by heat, postural change, or other mechanical or external influences.

## Headache

Headache must be analyzed precisely with particular reference to (1) its nature: whether deep or superficial, severe or mild, throbbing or aching, constant or intermittent; (2) its location, whether focal or generalized, unilateral or bilateral; (3) its incidence, whether periodic or regular in appearance; (4) the presence of associated ocular, neurologic, or systemic manifestations; (5) the factors that may precipitate or aggravate the headache, such as anxiety, changes in posture, ingestion of alcohol, or medication; and (6) those factors or agents that can be identified as providing relief.

## Seizures

A story of seizures requires precise elaboration. (1) It is important to determine the nature of the seizure itself, with particular reference to such features as the aura, if any, and the presence of generalized or focal characteristics during the overt attack. With major, generalized, attacks, such information may be obtainable only from relatives or friends, since the patient himself is usually unaware of such features. On the other hand, many features of petit mal or other minor attacks, motor or sensory jacksonian seizures, or uncinate and psychomotor episodes can commonly be recalled and described by the patient. (2) The association with loss or impairment of consciousness should be assessed. This is an extremely important factor, one on which depend important decisions relative to diagnosis, and one which must always be inquired about specifically. Falling during an attack, or tongue biting and/or incontinence may be of analagous significance. (3) The presence of postictal signs, particularly those of lateralizing quality, such as hemiparesis (Todd's paralysis), should be noted. (4) The occurrence of the attacks in terms of time should be clarified; for example, whether they occur chiefly during the day or in sleep, whether they develop in relationship to meals or to hunger, whether they appear related to fatigue or excitement and whether there would appear to be some temporal relationship to the menses. The spacing of attacks and their frequency must also be determined. (5) The onset of the attacks in a chronological sense must be established. It is vital to know whether attacks have been present from birth or whether they first became manifest during infancy, puberty, or adulthood. Changes in seizure pattern with the passage of years must be documented. Inquiry should be made into onset in relation to recognizable factors, such as head injury, infection, or stroke. (6) The response of the seizures to medication should be determined. A knowledge of the nature of drugs already utilized and their efficacy is of course helpful in planning rational therapy henceforth.

## Vertigo

Yet another common complaint requiring careful documentation is that of dizziness. Most patients, even those of good intelligence, do not really mean true vertigo when they complain of dizziness. It therefore becomes necessary to determine whether true subjective or objective vertigo is in fact present. The former consists of a sensation of movement or rotation of the patient himself; the latter comprises movement, or perhaps distortion, of objects in the environment. Ancillary symptoms of ataxia, nausea, or vomiting should be sought, since their presence supports the contention of true vertigo. Many patients use the term dizziness to indicate only a sensation of faintness, giddiness, or light-headedness, symptoms which are of much less specific connotation in a diagnostic sense. Careful questioning of the patient who describes dizziness should be repaid by a much clearer conception of the fundamental nature of the underlying disease process.

## Numbness

It is necessary to define as precisely as possible what is meant by the term numbness when used by any individual patient. In many instances it will be clear that weakness is meant, rather than true impairment or loss of sensation. The noting of paresthesia, often tingling in quality, may be of material assistance in clarifying the complaint. At times, patients complain of girdling sensations, or of feeling a limb encased in tight bandages or overly tight shoes, or of walking on air or on a pebbly surface; these variegated and often colorful symptoms are also of benefit in defining the true nature of a subjective sensation of numbness, since phenomena of this sort are experienced by individuals who have lesions involving especially the posterior column sensory system. Curiously, many patients with bona fide sensory defects involving spinothalamic modalities of sensation may be themselves totally unaware of this shortcoming and, thus, proffer no spontaneous symptoms in this regard. Finally, one must determine whether a complaint of numbness has developed simultaneously throughout the affected part, or whether it has progressed from one part of the limb to another, as epitomized, for example, by a sensory jacksonian march.

## Visual Abnormality

A complaint of blurring of vision may actually mean any one of a variety of alterations of vision and must be looked into carefully. It may mean exactly what it suggests, but it may also refer to phenomena as diverse as double vision, indistinct vision due to a scotoma, loss of vision associated with a hemianopic field defect, distortion of vision as encountered in migraine, or simply reduced visual acuity. These can and should be distinguished by proper questioning. Diplopia especially must be analyzed to determine if true double vision is present. If so, the position of the objects in relationship to one another should be determined and, if possible, the identity of the false image established. When diplopia is monocular, a diagnosis of hysteria suggests itself, but monocular diplopia may in fact be observed in instances of local ocular disease such as dislocation of the lens or retinal separation. Ancillary symptoms such as ocular pain, particularly on movement of the globe, defects in color vision, and related neurologic symptoms must of course always be sought in the patient with visual impairment.

The foregoing are samples of the method of inquiry required to analyze specific symptoms presented by patients suffering from a neurologic disorder. They serve to emphasize the central fact that no history can be accepted at face value; all symptoms must be analyzed carefully and extensively in order to achieve an accurate diagnosis. The importance of such a precise evaluation should not be underestimated. The fact that the great majority of neurologic diagnoses are actually made on the basis of the history underscores the importance of such a thorough and searching analysis, a classic approach that continues to underlie the practice of clinical neurology today.

## Additional Historical Features

When the history of the *present illness* has been completed, details of the occupational, social, and past medical histories must be uncovered to determine whether these offer clues of importance. Not only must environmental factors such as exposure to lead, arsenic, carbon disulfide, organic mercurials, insecticides, organic solvents, cold, and other hazards be investigated, but it is equally important to determine the presence of occupational tension and stress. The quality of the patient's adjustment to the work and home environment must be defined. The pertinence of the past medical history will of course depend on the specific nature of the illnesses from which the patient has suffered. Abuse of alcohol and of a variety of other drugs should be sought. The educational history may also be helpful, especially when the question of intellectual deterioration has been raised.

No history can be regarded as complete without at least limited inquiry into the patient's personality structure. Illness invariably evokes some degree of anxiety, which in turn is responsible for the development of reactions that may obscure the basic symptoms of the structural illness. Such reactions may in some instances become so pronounced as to dominate the entire clinical picture. It is therefore important to assess the premorbid personality and behavioral patterns of the person who has developed the illness being probed. For this purpose a brief personality survey must be made. An appraisal of the patient's personality structure that covers feelings, attitudes, goals, and frustrations is useful. Diverse factors such as the patient's relationship to other members of the family and his or her marital adjustment should be assessed.

Finally, information as to handedness should be sought in an attempt to determine the laterality of cerebral dominance. This is of particular importance when one is dealing with patients suffering from disorders of language and other higher integrative functions. The question as to which eye and which foot are predominant may also merit investigation, as well as family patterns of dexterity and dominance.

The main features of the history having been determined, the patient is then ready for examination.

# THE NEUROLOGIC EXAMINATION

## Consciousness and Mentation

First, and most importantly, the state of awareness (i.e., of consciousness and of responsiveness) must be determined. If altered, the precise nature and degree of impairment should be defined (see Chapter 2 for a detailed description of abnormalities encountered and their putative significance). Particularly in the conscious and alert patient, the physician is offered at the outset an opportunity to study various features of importance. The facial expression should be noted, and such features as facial mobility and anxiety, appearance of depression or dejection, asymmetries of movement, and presence of abnormal movements observed. The general intellectual level of the patient and his premorbid attainment may be roughly estimated by the richness or poverty of his *vocabulary,* by the manner of presentation of the historical material, by the occupational background, and by the general pattern of activity. Responses to questions concerning general *fund of knowledge* and culture also shed light on the intellectual background, at least in a formal educational sense.

It is generally possible at the bedside to determine whether there are signs of intellectual impairment and whether there is clouding of the sensorium (Table 1-1). If an intellectual deficit (i.e., *dementia*) is in fact found, formal psychologic testing may be of considerable value in measuring the extent of the deficit. However, with relatively simple testing one can acquire a remarkably sophisticated appraisal of the patient's cognitive performance without such formal evaluation. It should be emphasized that loss of intellectual function is usually the result of structural brain disease; however, slowing of intellectual processes *(bradyphrenia)* may be found in depressed, anxious, or severely distracted individuals. The thought disorders of the schizophrenic may mimic those of the individual with organic brain disease. At times it is difficult to distinguish the congenitally retarded person from the patient with an acquired intellectual deficit; under such circumstances, formal psychologic testing may be of particular assistance.

Early in the course of the examination the patient's *orientation* for time, place, and person should be determined. *Memory* for events of both the recent and remote past can and should be tested, often during the course of the history-taking itself. Efforts should be made to determine dates of birth, marriage, graduation from school, and other pertinent data. Recent recall can be assessed by asking when and how the patient came to the hospital, by asking him to recall the name of his physician and his own address, and by determining his ability to give an adequate account

**TABLE 1-1.** Evaluation of the mental status

| |
|---|
| ATTENTION SPAN (Digit Retention) |
| ORIENTATION |
| Time |
| Place |
| Person |
| MEMORY |
| Immediate Recall (Digit Retention) |
| Recent (Series of Test Objects) |
| Remote |
| FUND OF GENERAL KNOWLEDGE |
| CALCULATION (Serial 7's) |
| ABSTRACT THINKING |
| Proverb Explanation |
| Similarities |
| JUDGMENT, INSIGHT |
| MOOD, BEHAVIOR |
| OTHER |
| Personal and/or Spatial Inattention |
| Design Copying |
| Projective Drawing |

of his own illness. Alternatively, the patient may be presented with a simple story and asked to repeat it, or requested to memorize and subsequently recall several items such as the name of a flower or a hypothetical street address. Test sentences designed to avoid emotional coloration, for example, "There is one thing a nation needs to be strong and great and that is a firm, secure supply of wood," are sometimes used for this purpose as well. The *attention span,* vital to such tests of memory, is evaluated during the give and take of the history; it may be investigated more formally by tests of *digit retention,* which appraise the ability of the patient to repeat series of digits forward and backward. When digits are presented at an even rate of one per second, without recognizable rhythm or grouping, the normal adult can recall and repeat approximately five, six, or more digits forward, and four or five in reverse. As mentioned above, the *fund of general information* should be tested by inquiring, for example, after the names of the presidents, past and present, the governor of the state, the capital of states and countries, important dates, outstanding items of current events, or sports results.

The ability to *calculate* must be tested routinely. The serial seven test is most commonly employed for this purpose, with the patient being requested to subtract 7 beginning with 100 (100 − 7, 93 − 7, etc.). Other simple arithmetic problems can be tested (e.g., the number of inches in 3 3/4 feet; if 5 times × equals 20, how much is ×). In patients with a limited educational background, calculations such as these may be *a priori* impossible, and more mundane arithmetic devices such as a grocery shopping list should be employed. Since a shift from the abstract to the concrete attitude in thought may be a very sensitive indicator of a dementing process, the ability to think in the *abstract* must also be determined. This can be evaluated by asking the patient to explain common proverbs ("People who live in glass houses shouldn't throw stones," "A bird in the hand is worth two in the bush," "Don't cry over spilled milk"), or to determine similarities in classes of objects ("Why is a cat like a lion?"). Again, those with an impoverished formal education and few day-to-day intellectual demands may think much more concretely than would ordinarily be anticipated. As previously indicated, an attempt should be made to assess the *premorbid intellectual attainment* of the patient by determining the level of available *vocabulary,* since this function commonly appears most resistant to impairment in the course of illnesses characterized by progressive intellectual failure.

Attention must also be directed toward other higher integrative and neuropsychologic functions. *Speech* and *language* can generally be assessed during the course of the history-taking, and it should be determined whether dysarthria, aphasia, or other derangement of communication is present (see Chapter 2). In appropriate cases it may be necessary to utilize specific language testing, directed, for example, toward the patient's ability to express himself fluently and in an effective manner, to comprehend and respond to verbal symbols (language) of increasing complexity, and to recognize, name, and demonstrate the appropriate use of various objects. In patients with relatively mild disorders of expressive or receptive language, or both, ordinary communication may not be grossly deranged, and correct identification of the defect may be possible only with such specific testing. The ability to read and write must also be evaluated; again, tasks of increasing complexity may be utilized in both spheres. The integrity of the *body scheme,* or image, must also be determined. Awareness of the relationships of one part of the body to another, and of the body to extracorporeal space, must be noted, as well as the ability to conceptualize spatial relationships in a normal fashion. When indicated, specific testing with drawings (such as of the face of a clock or a flower), with design copying and completion, and with construction of figures with matchsticks and varicolored cubes may be employed.

Efforts must also be made to determine impairment of *judgment.* The history may provide vital data in this respect. Judgment may be further assessed by the patient's pattern of response to standard test questions, for example, "What would you do if you smelled smoke in a crowded theater?" Changes in personality and the degree of a patient's insight into his illness must also be established. The presence of delusions, hallucinations, obsessions, and phobias must be investigated in appropriate instances. The *mood* and general reaction of the patient to his illness should of course be observed during the examination, and the presence of anxiety, depression, excitement, suspicion, and the like documented when encountered.

# The Cranial Nerves

## OLFACTORY (I)

The olfactory nerve does not require detailed investigation for routine purposes; evaluation of its function is especially pertinent in instances of trauma, and in patients with visual failure or progressive intellectual deterioration. It is examined by alternately occluding the patient's nostrils and asking him to smell substances such as coffee, cloves, or lemon extract with the open nostril. A patent airway is of course essential for accurate testing. Other aromatic substances such as tobacco, peppermint, or vinegar may be utilized; highly volatile substances such as ammonia should be avoided. Distinction between odors is more important than precise identification of any given substance.

## OPTIC (II)

The optic nerve is directly examined by means of an ophthalmoscope and tested by investigation of the visual acuity and the visual fields. Every physician should naturally become skilled in the use of an ophthalmoscope, since information of great value can be obtained from the fundus oculi in a variety of circumstances. The visual acuity is tested most simply by means of readily available standardized charts. When these are not at hand, acuity may be determined crudely by assessing the ability of the patient to read various sizes of newsprint, or by counting fingers, or, in the face of severe visual handicap, by the ability to distinguish between light and darkness. Corrective lenses should be worn in order to determine the best corrected visual acuity. When these are not available to overcome refractive errors, the patient should be asked to look through a pin-hole or a series of pin-holes, since this technique compensates for a refractive error to a considerable extent. Color vision may be evaluated in patients with visual failure, preferably utilizing the standard Ishihara plates.

For complete study, the visual fields (Fig. 1-2) must be examined by means of a perimeter and a tangent screen. However, gross visual field defects may be detected by means of confrontation. The patient faces the examiner at a distance of two or three feet, covers one eye with his hand, and fixes his gaze on the examiner's nose or facing eye. The patient's degree of fixation may thus be monitored directly by the examiner during testing. The examiner's finger is then brought in along the main axes of the visual field, preferably at 45° intervals around the full circle; the patient calls out as soon as the finger is seen. A long pin with a white head may be used for more accurate determinations. On occasion, colored test objects, particularly red ones, prove useful. The relative brightness of a colored test object in various portions of a monocular field may prove particularly helpful in identifying a scotoma or hemianopic defect. In instances of

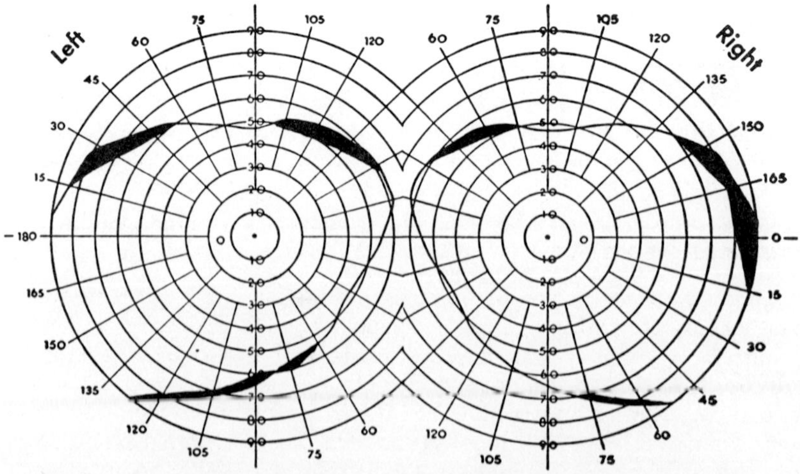


**FIGURE 1-2.** Normal visual fields showing the characteristic flattening above and on the nasal sides. By convention, fields are recorded as the patient sees them, that is, with the right eye (OD) on the right, the left (OS) on the left.

severe visual loss, the fields may be mapped out by means of a flashlight. With appropriate utilization of the confrontation method, both hemianopic field defects and scotomas are generally detected without difficulty. Indeed, with a cooperative patient even the relative size of the blind spot can be determined in this manner. During testing of the visual fields, stimuli should also be exposed simultaneously in both halves of the field; if this is not done, an attention visual defect, as found, for example, in patients with parietal lobe lesions, may escape recognition. In stuporous patients, the response to a threatening stimulus on either side may be used as a very crude guide to the integrity of the visual fields.

## OCULOMOTOR (III), TROCHLEAR (IV), ABDUCENS (VI)

The nerves concerned with ocular and pupillary motility are most simply examined together.

### Pupillary Reflex

This reflex is tested preferably in darkness or shade, by flashing a light in the pupil while examining the size, regularity, shape, and reaction in response to the stimulus. Normally the pupils are equal in size and regular in outline. Under ordinary circumstances the pupil reacts promptly to direct light, the contraction being maintained for a very brief time and then relaxing as the sphincter of the iris fatigues with continued application of the light. The consensual response (i.e., the contraction of the pupil opposite to that directly stimulated by the light) should also be observed. The testing light should also be swung rapidly back and forth between both eyes, searching for the paradoxical dilatation of a denervated pupil (Marcus Gunn pupil). Finally, the accommodation reflex should be tested by observing the size of the pupil as it accommodates to near and far vision. At times, the response of the pupil to various pharmacologic agents must be determined (this is discussed more fully in Chapter 2).

## Ocular Movements

Conjugate movements are tested by asking the patient to look voluntarily to either side or vertically, as far as possible, and to follow a moving finger or light. Convergence is tested by asking the patient to look at the finger at a distance and on close inspection. Individual eye movements are appraised by covering one eye and observing movement of the other in all axes. When evaluating individual extraocular muscles, care must be taken to avoid movements that utilize several muscles simultaneously; each muscle should be tested in its position of maximal action (Figs. 1-3 and 1-4). Limitation of movement is looked for. The patient must always be queried as to the occurrence of double vision. When a complaint of diplopia is elicited, the site of maximal separation of images must be determined in an attempt to define the specific muscular paresis responsible for the complaint. This is sometimes expedited by the red glass test. One eye is covered with a piece of red glass or plastic, and the patient is asked to follow a moving light with both eyes open; this technique permits quick and accurate delineation of defective ocular movement by breaking up the images derived from the two eyes into differently colored and, thus, easily distinguished objects. This maneuver may permit a latent squint to become manifest, and results must be interpreted with care.

During testing of ocular motility, the presence or absence of nystagmus, and its characteristics, should be noted. Opticokinetic nystagmus may be evaluated by observing the pattern of ocular response in reaction to the movements of a striped tape or drum positioned in front of the

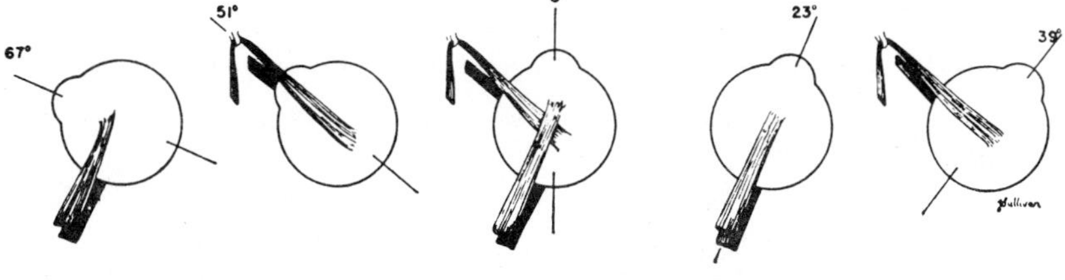


**FIGURE 1-3.** Diagram illustrating the positions and actions of the vertical recti and oblique muscles in different positions of gaze of the right eye; the medial and lateral recti, which act solely as adductor or abductor of the globe respectively, are not indicated. (From Cogan, D.: *Neurology of the Ocular Muscles.* ed. 2, 1963. Courtesy of Charles C Thomas, Publisher, Springfield, Ill.)

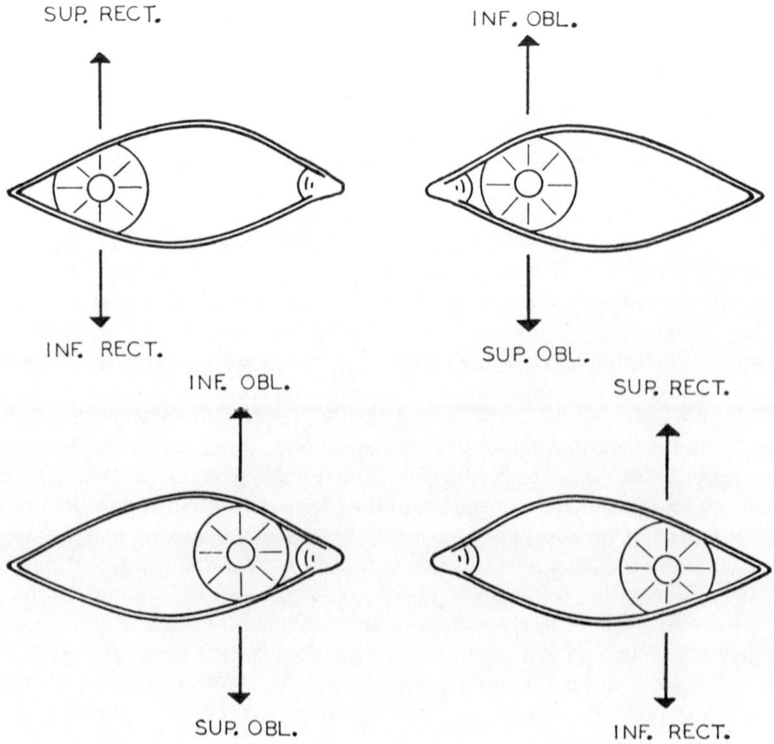


**FIGURE 1-4.** Diagram indicating the muscles chiefly responsible for vertical movements of the eyes in different positions of gaze. (From Cogan, D.: *Neurology of the Ocular Muscles.* ed. 2, 1963. Courtesy of Charles C Thomas, Publisher, Springfield, Ill.)

patient's eyes. The patient's fixation and cooperation are important factors in the elicitation of normal opticokinetic responses, overcome to some extent by using a very broad stimulus.

## TRIGEMINAL (V)

The *motor* component of this nerve is tested by asking the patient to clench his teeth and to chew, with the examiner feeling the masseter and temporal muscles directly to determine both the force of contraction and muscle bulk. The pterygoids may be tested by having the patient compress the jaw laterally against the examiner's finger, with the mouth being held partially open. Deviation of the jaw caused by masseter paralysis is demonstrated by asking the patient to open the mouth and noting that the jaw deviates to the weak side. The *sensory* portion of the trigeminal nerve is evaluated by testing facial sensibility and the corneal reflex. The latter is extremely important under some circumstances, but as ordinarily elicited it has little value since most often it is brought out not by stimulation of the cornea but of the sclera. It should be tested in such a manner that the stimulus is invisible to the patient, who will naturally blink on seeing an object approach the eye. A fine hair mounted on an applicator, or a teased-out wisp of cotton, can stimulate the cornea directly without being seen by the patient. The normal response consists of a rapid, forceful contraction of the eyelid similar to that experienced when a foreign body enters the eye. A contralateral blink is characteristic. When the presence of a facial paralysis interferes with the efferent (i.e., motor) portion of the reflex, the afferent component may be evaluated by observing particularly this contralateral response. The patient should be queried as to whether the stimulus itself has been felt as well. Facial sensation is evaluated by testing the skin of the face for the ability to perceive pain, thermal sensation, and light touch. As with most other aspects of the neurologic examination, this is always performed by comparing one side of the face with the other. The mucous membranes of the nose, the mouth, and the anterior portion of the tongue may also be tested in this manner. On occasion, it is useful to evaluate the proprioceptive function of the trigeminal nerve, utilizing particularly the earlobe for this purpose. It should be borne in mind that different central trigeminal pathways subserve different sensory modalities over the face. Thus, appreciation of pain is mediated via the spinal nucleus and tract of the trigeminal, whereas touch is represented in the principle sensory nucleus and tract, and proprioception in the mesencephalic root. At times valuable information as to localization of a brainstem lesion may be derived from the recognition of differential patterns of sensory impairment in the trigeminal distribution.

## FACIAL (VII)

Both upper and lower divisions of the facial nerve should be tested routinely. The patient is asked to wrinkle the forehead and to frown (frontalis muscle), to close the eyelids tightly or to wink (orbicularis oculi), and to open the mouth, retract the mouth, blow out the cheeks, pucker the lips, screw up the nose, whistle, and so on (orbicularis oris and other muscles of facial expression). By these maneuvers the several muscles innervated by the facial nerve are tested and the presence and distribution of weakness are easily detected. It will be recalled that in addition to innervating the musculature of the face, the facial nerve also supplies taste fibers to the anterior two thirds of the tongue via the lingual nerve. This need not be tested routinely, but in instances of peripheral facial paralysis (e.g., Bell's palsy), it becomes necessary to determine whether the taste fibers are in fact involved. This may be tested by having the patient protrude the tongue and applying substances such as sugar, salt, and quinine. The patient is asked to detect the substance used without retracting the tongue, generally an easy performance for the normal subject.

## AUDITORY (VIII)

Both cochlear and vestibular portions of the auditory nerve are examined.

### Cochlear

This portion is concerned with hearing and may be tested crudely by observing the patient's ability to hear a spoken voice or a whisper. It can also be tested by simple tuning fork procedures using a fork of 512 cps or higher (Rinne test). The fork is placed in vibration on the mastoid process, and the patient asked to inform the examiner when the vibration has ceased. At this point the fork is placed next to the ear and the patient asked whether the tuning fork can still be heard. Under normal circumstances, air conduction (AC) is greater than bone conduction (BC), and the fork will be heard here after it is no longer heard on the bone itself. Measurement may be made of the time over which the tuning fork is heard over the bone as compared with air, but for routine purposes this is not necessary. In nerve deafness, both air and bone conduction may be reduced, but the normal formula (AC > BC) pertains. On the other hand, in conduction deafness bone conduction is better than air. Lateralization tests are also utilized (Weber test). A tuning fork is placed on the forehead, and with one ear completely occluded by the examiner's finger the patient is asked to indicate on which side the vibration is loudest. It is normally heard best on the occluded side. In conduction deafness the tuning fork is referred to the diseased ear, whereas in nerve deafness it cannot be heard on the affected side. For more precise examination of audition, detailed audiometric evaluation is required.

### Vestibular

This portion of the nerve is tested in a variety of ways. One is the past-pointing test. The patient is asked to raise his arm and to bring the index finger down onto the examiner's finger with the arm outstretched, first with the eyes open, then closed. Normally the patient's finger touches the examiner's without difficulty, whereas in vestibular disease the finger past-points to one side or the other. Past-pointing may also be noted in such tests as the finger-to-nose maneuver. The patient with disease of the vestibular portion of the VIII nerve may also exhibit ataxia of the trunk or of the limbs, generally in association with a complaint of vertigo, at times sufficiently severe to be confused with cerebellar dysfunction.

The function of the vestibular portion of the auditory nerve is also evaluated at least in part by a search for nystagmus. The nystagmus of vestibular or labyrinthine affection is a rhythmic movement of the eyeballs with slow and fast components, and is either horizontal or rotary in character. The fast movement is to the side of ocular deviation; the slow movement is a compensatory return to the midline. At times nystagmus in the vertical plane is also encountered. (A detailed discussion of nystagmus is found in Chapter 2.)

At the bedside, *caloric* testing is simply done and may prove remarkably informative, particularly in the evaluation of the comatose patient. This consists of stimulation of the semicircular canals by the instillation of cold water (18° to 20°C) slowly into the external canal with the patient recumbent and the head elevated to approximately 30°. Following introduction of such cold water, observations are made as to (1) nystagmus, (2) past-pointing, and (3) development of vertigo, nausea, or vomiting. When the patient's head is elevated, the vertical canals are stimulated; the responses of the horizontal canals may be tested by flexing the head forward. After irrigation of the ears with ice water, a well-established pattern of normal responses may be observed. Thus, after irrigation of the right ear, one notes (1) vertigo developing within 2 minutes of beginning of irrigation; (2) mixed lateral and rotary nystagmus to the left; (3) past-pointing to the right; (4) nausea and at times vomiting; (5) increase of nystagmus to the right side with the head flexed; and (6) intensification of vertigo, nystagmus, and past-pointing on return of the head to the upright position. After irrigation of the left ear, the subjective reactions such as nausea, vomiting, and vertigo remain the same, but nystagmus is to the right and past-pointing chiefly to the left. Other more sophisticated tests of vestibular function, such as electronystagmography, are helpful under certain circumstances. Alterations of caloric responses are found in a wide variety of circumstances. In cerebellopontine angle tumors, for example, an absence of response may be noted on the side of the tumor or, in other instances, a perversion of responses with nystagmus occurring to the wrong side may be noted. Patients with intrinsic disease of the brainstem may exhibit alterations in the pattern of caloric response; in patients in deep coma, loss of the caloric responses has a grave prognostic significance. Altered responses may also be encountered in patients with end-organ (e.g., labyrinthine) disease.

## GLOSSOPHARYNGEAL (IX)

This nerve is tested routinely with the vagus. Its chief function is sensory, supplying particularly the pharynx. Taste over the posterior third of the tongue is mediated through the glossopharyngeal nerve as well. The only motor function of the nerve concerns movement of the pharynx by means of the stylopharyngeus muscle, a role so minor as to be virtually untestable.

## VAGUS (X)

The vagus nerve is the principle motor nerve of the pharynx and larynx. It is tested routinely by observing pharyngeal movements, most simply by asking the patient to phonate by saying "Ah." Normally the soft palate and uvula elevate in the midline. With weakness of one side, the palate deviates upwards on phonation to the healthy side, while the diseased side droops; in cases of bilateral paralysis no palatal movements are observed. The pharyngeal (gag) reflex is tested by stimulating the back of the pharynx with a throat stick and observing the ensuing and normally symmetrical contraction of the palatal muscles. Since the vocal cords are also supplied through the vagus, by the recurrent laryngeal nerve, assessment of the timbre of the voice is an essential part of the evaluation of vagal function. In instances of hoarseness or aphonia, laryngoscopy, direct or indirect, is advisable.

It is difficult to assess the autonomic functions of the vagus nerve during a routine examination.

## SPINAL ACCESSORY (XI)

This nerve innervates the trapezius and sternomastoid muscles. The function of the former is tested by asking the patient to shrug the shoulders against resistance, and of the latter by turning the head against resistance. Both sternomastoids may be tested simultaneously by having the patient flex his head forcefully against a resisting hand.

## HYPOGLOSSAL (XII)

Function of this, the motor nerve of the tongue, is most simply tested by asking the patient to protrude the tongue. Under normal circumstances, the tongue protrudes in the midline. In paralysis of the tongue caused by affection of the nerve there is deviation to the paretic side. Strength of the tongue may be assessed directly by asking the patient to press the tongue against the cheek, thrusting against the examiner's fingers. Atrophy and involuntary movements of the tongue are ordinarily apparent with simple inspection; recognition of fasciculations requires that the tongue be at rest in the floor of the mouth, since many normal individuals exhibit tremulousness of the tongue when it is extended. The ability to maintain the tongue in a protruded position should also be assessed; in some disorders, such as Huntington's disease, the tongue cannot be maintained in such a position, but darts back and forth in a serpentine manner.

For ordinary routine purposes in a busy general practice, examination of the visual fields, pupillary reflexes, ocular movements, facial innervation, and movements of the pharynx and tongue are the most important aspects of the cranial nerve examination, supplemented by an accurate funduscopic appraisal. Whenever possible, and certainly when indicated by specific symptoms, a more thorough examination of all cranial nerve functions is naturally desirable.

## MOTOR SYSTEM

Examination of the motor system includes the determination of *muscle power, bulk,* and *tone,* observation of the occurrence of *involuntary movements* such as fasciculations and tremors, and an assessment of the status of the muscle stretch *reflexes.* Evaluation of *cerebellar function* may also be considered within the general scope of this part of the examination. As with other aspects of the neurologic examination, rigorous comparison of one side of the body with the other is vital, the patient serving as his or her own control. For the routine determination of weakness or strength of muscles, a few simple maneuvers are ordinarily sufficient; more detailed evaluation may be carried out as prompted by the clinical presentation in any given patient. (See Appendix for tables of innervation of muscles.)

### Muscle Power

#### UPPER EXTREMITIES

A sampling of both proximal and distal muscles should be routine. The hand grips are tested by asking the patient to squeeze the examiner's fingers; inquiry as to whether the patient is right- or left-handed may be helpful. The power of the hand grip may be assessed by the force required to withdraw the fingers from the clenched fist. The patient is also asked to fix the tightly clenched fist at the wrist, with the examiner attempting to overcome such maximal dorsiflexion. It is virtually impossible to overcome wrist dorsiflexion in normal individuals except, perhaps, for the very young or the elderly; this then becomes an especially useful gauge of strength, subject to little individual variation. Abduction of the fingers against resistance, and opposition of the thumb, may also be tested simply and quickly. More proximal strength is evaluated by asking the patient to flex and extend the forearm against resistance and to abduct the arms at the shoulders. Under appropriate circumstances, for example, when there is a history of neck, shoulder, or arm pain, much more detailed examination of the muscles of the shoulder girdle, arms, and hands is required. The relatively simple testing described does however provide a rapid and reasonably accurate appraisal of the motor function of the principle peripheral nerves supplying the upper extremities.

#### LOWER EXTREMITIES

Once again, both proximal and distal strength must be investigated. Distal strength in the lower extremities is most simply tested by evaluating dorsiflexion of the feet; the patient is requested to dorsiflex the foot forcefully against the examiner's hand. Plantar flexion is tested by pushing down against the hand. Dorsiflexion and plantar flexion of the feet may also be evaluated by observing the patient's ability to walk on the heels and on the toes. More proximally, the power of extension and flexion of the leg at the knee, and at the hip, should also be determined. As in the arms, symptoms may suggest more detailed testing of muscle power.

## Muscle Tone

While the musculature is being examined for evidence of weakness, *muscle tone* should also be investigated. A determination of tone is based on the examiner's judgment as to the degree and quality of resistance to passive movements of the limbs at selected joints, most commonly the fingers, wrists, elbows, and knees. In light of the considerable variation in tone in normal individuals, caution must be exercised in the interpretation of apparent abnormalities. Changes such as flaccidity, spasticity, or rigidity must be identified and the distribution of such alterations (i.e., whether focal, lateralized, or generalized) established. In the very young, in the elderly, in dements, and in some psychotic individuals, the phenomenon of *paratonia* (gegenhalten) may give rise to a spurious impression of heightened muscle tone and must be watched for carefully. This abnormality, appearing promptly when the limb is grasped by the examiner, involves all the muscles in the limb equally. It may at times be difficult to separate from true hypertonicity; when the patient's spontaneous movements are observed surreptitiously, however, no restriction of motility can be seen, a feature helpful at times in drawing this distinction.

## Muscle Bulk

The *bulk* of the muscles also requires evaluation. Muscle atrophy should be searched for, and, if found, its distribution determined. Fasciculations should always be looked for, whether or not atrophy is present. An increase in muscle bulk may be observed in some individuals, at times associated with increased strength (as in work hypertrophy), and at other times with reduced power, as in the so-called pseudohypertrophy encountered in some instances of muscular dystrophy.

Throughout the course of the motor examination, the presence of *involuntary movements* such as chorea, athetosis or dystonia, tremors, tics, myoclonic jerks, or other adventitious movements should be noted.

To one who is well versed in the routine examination of the nervous system, all this and more can be carried out quickly and accurately in assessment of the motor apparatus. For routine purposes in which the neurologic examination is part of a general physical survey of the patient, evaluation may be restricted to a determination of power in selected proximal and distal muscles in all limbs, observation for involuntary movements, and assessment of the state of reflex activity and coordination of the limbs.

## REFLEXES (Table 1-2)

### Jaw Jerk

This reflex is obtained by tapping the chin briskly when the mouth is held partially open. The normal response is a rapid closure of the jaw. A heightened briskness of response is sought. Not often tested, this reflex may be of substantial value in determining the segmental level of a lesion in a patient exhibiting bilateral pyramidal tract signs.

### Biceps Reflex

The biceps reflex is examined by placing the elbow of the arm being tested in the hand of the examiner, with the examiner's thumb being placed over the biceps tendon and struck briskly with a reflex hammer. The anticipated result is flexion of the forearm.

### Brachioradial Reflex

This reflex is elicited by tapping the lower third of the radius with the forearm placed midway between pronation and supination. The normal response is flexion of the forearm on the arm and, usually, flexion of the fingers and hand as well. Often neglected, this is an extremely useful reflex to assess. With a lesion in the fifth cervical segment, tapping the radius may cause flexion only of the hand and the fingers, but not of the forearm, which may in fact extend (inversion of the radial reflex); a similar

**TABLE 1-2.** Important muscle stretch reflexes

| | ELICITED BY | RESPONSE | SEGMENTAL LEVEL |
|---|---|---|---|
| JAW | Tapping mandible in half-open position | Closure of jaw | Pons |
| SCAPULO-HUMERAL | Tapping vertebral border of scapula | Contraction of teres minor, infraspinatus, etc. | C5 and C6 |
| TRICEPS | Tapping triceps tendon | Extension at elbow | C7 to D1 |
| BICEPS | Tapping biceps tendon | Flexion at elbow | C5 and C6 |
| RADIAL | Tapping syloid process of radius | Contraction of supinator longus | C5 and C6 |
| KNEE | Tapping patellar tendon | Extension at knee | L3 and L4 |
| ANKLE | Tapping Achilles tendon | Extension at ankle | S1 and S2 |

response, however, may occasionally be noted in some normal individuals, and in instances of myopathy.

## Triceps Reflex

The patient's arm is supported under the elbow and partially extended; the triceps tendon is tapped by the reflex hammer. Extension of the forearm results. In the supine position, the arm is positioned across the chest with the forearm slightly flexed, and the triceps tendon is tapped just above the olecranon.

## Patellar Reflex

The patellar tendon of the partially extended leg is tapped. If sought for with the patient in bed, placing a rolled pillow under the knees facilitates the reflex activity.

## Achilles Reflex

This reflex may be demonstrated in a variety of ways. With the patient lying on his face (prone), the knee is flexed and the foot held slightly dorsiflexed by the examiner's hand; the Achilles tendon is then struck, resulting normally in plantar flexion. Alternatively, the patient may kneel on a chair while the Achilles tendon is struck, or he may lie on his back with legs flexed and everted, the Achilles tendon being percussed while the foot is held dorsiflexed.

## Plantar Reflex

For routine purposes the sole of the foot is stimulated by a fairly blunt object such as a key carried along the outer margin of the foot and then across the ball. The normal response is flexion of the toes.

## Superficial Reflexes

A number of superficial reflexes may be elicited (Table 1–3). Among these, the *abdominal reflexes* are perhaps the most useful. These are obtained by drawing an object, such as the blunt end of a stick, a pin, key, or brush, along the upper and lower abdominal quadrants on either side. A normal response comprises contraction of the abdominal musculature and resultant pull of the umbilicus toward the stimulated side. Maximal relaxation of the abdominal muscles is essential for satisfactory testing; when the muscles have been unduly stretched, as by repeated pregnancies, the abdominal reflexes may be difficult or impossible to obtain. The *cremasteric reflexes* are also easily demonstrated. These are elicited by stimulating the inner side of the thigh, retraction of the ipsilateral testicle representing a normal response.

**TABLE 1-3.** Important superficial reflexes

| | ELICITED BY | RESPONSE | SEGMENTAL LEVEL |
|---|---|---|---|
| CORNEAL | Touching cornea with hair | Contraction of orbicularis oculi | Pons |
| PHARYNGEAL | Touching posterior wall of pharynx | Contraction of pharynx | Medulla |
| PALATAL | Touching soft palate | Elevation of palate | Medulla |
| SCAPULAR | Stroking skin between scapulae | Contraction of scapular muscles | C5 to D1 |
| EPIGASTRIC | Stroking downward from nipples | Dimpling of epigastrium ipsilaterally | D7 to D9 |
| ABDOMINAL | Stroking beneath costal margins and above inguinal ligament | Contraction of abdominal muscles in quadrant stimulated | D8 to D12 |
| CREMASTERIC | Stroking medial surface of upper thigh | Ipsilateral elevation of testicle | L1 and L2 |
| GLUTEAL | Stroking skin of buttock | Contraction of glutei | L4 and L5 |
| BULBO-CAVERNOUS | Pinching dorsum of glans | Contraction of bulbous urethra | S3 and S4 |
| SUPERFICIAL ANAL | Pricking perineum | Contraction of rectal sphincters | S5 and coccygeal |

## Additional Reflexes

A variety of other muscle stretch reflexes may be sought when the clinical situation demands. The *orbicularis oculi reflex* is brought out as follows: the skin at the outer corner of the eye is held between the thumb and index finger and is pulled back slightly; the thumb is tapped lightly with a reflex hammer. A reflex contraction of the orbicularis oculi follows. Diminution of this reflex may be found in peripheral facial palsy, whereas the reflex is preserved in central facial palsies. The *scapulohumeral reflex* may be elicited by tapping the vertebral border of the scapula; contraction of the musculature of the shoulder girdle and abduction of the arm results therefrom. Many muscles are brought into play with this maneuver, particularly the deltoid, pectoralis major, infraspinatus, and teres minor. The reflex may be lost unilaterally with lesions in the fifth cervical segment. The *adductor reflex of the thigh* is obtained by placing the finger on the medial condyle of the femur with the legs slightly adducted. When the finger is tapped, adduction of the leg follows. At times, especially with pyramidal tract disease, crossed adduction also appears. The *biceps femoris reflex* is best elicited with the patient lying on the side opposite the one being examined, with the leg bent at the hip and knee. The finger is placed on the hamstring tendon and tapped with a hammer; contraction of the hamstring follows.

When the muscle stretch reflexes are difficult to obtain utilizing ordinary techniques, the patient is asked to clench or squeeze his hands together while the examiner attempts to elicit the reflex. This maneuver, termed *reinforcement,* may bring out reflexes not otherwise obtainable.

A number of other reflexes of varying degrees of complexity can be found that may be interpreted as representing a reversion to a primitive (i.e., infantile) level of reflex functioning. Thus, in some patients with cerebral hemispheral disease involving especially, although not exclusively, the frontal lobes, reflexes that are normally encountered only in infancy may make a reappearance. Among these are several perioral release phenomena, including the *snout reflex,* a pursing response of the lips to a brisk tap above or below the mouth, and visual and tactile *sucking,* elicited by approaching or touching the lips with a blunt object. In such patients, brisk stimulation of the palm of the hand with a noxious stimulus may result in a retraction of the perioral muscles on the same side, the *palmomental reflex.* Light tactile stimulation across the palm may induce *forced grasping,* a reflex response that may at times be confused with a voluntary grasp; in the reflex variety, the grasp becomes more powerful as the examiner attempts to withdraw his hand. In contrast to the grasp reflex, which is ordinarily taken as evidence of frontal disease, patients with parietal lobe disorder may demonstrate the opposite, that is, an *avoidance* response to much the same form of stimulus. Reflexes of this type are discussed further in Chapter 2.

## CEREBELLAR SYSTEM

A survey should routinely be made of the functioning of the cerebellum and its connections, with particular attention to the ability to coordinate movements into smooth and effectual patterns. Testing is directed both to the limbs and to the trunk. When evaluating the results of such tests, care must be taken to exclude proprioceptive defects and weakness, either of which may lead to confusion in interpretation.

For ordinary purposes the finger-nose, heel-knee, and pronation-supination tests, as well as evaluation of the gait and station, will provide key information as to cerebellar function and will generally suffice for this end.

## Upper Extremities

### FINGER-NOSE TEST

The patient is asked to place the index finger of either hand on the nose. This is normally performed smoothly and easily with eyes both open and closed. The test may be varied by asking the patient to touch the nose in rapid succession several times.

### FINGER-FINGER TEST

The patient places his index finger on the examiner's index, generally several times in rapid succession with eyes both open and closed.

### PRONATION-SUPINATION TEST

With the arms extended in front of him, the patient is asked to pronate and supinate rapidly using the elbows as a fulcrum. Normally, the movements are of equal amplitude, smooth and even, with a well-maintained rhythm. The arms should not drift during the performance of this test.

### PATTING TEST

The patient is asked to pat rapidly the examiner's hand or his own thigh. Under normal conditions this is performed briskly with even amplitude and rhythm.

### REBOUND TEST

The ability to check movements quickly, which requires the coordinated action of agonists, antagonists, and synergists, especially around large joints, is tested by observing the response to sudden passive displacement of the outstretched arms. Normally, such a movement is rapidly checked, with the displaced limb returning to its initial position evenly and accurately.

### DEXTERITY TEST

Dexterity of the hands is evaluated by asking the patient to perform fine movements such as rapidly touching the fingertips with the thumb in sequential fashion. This is normally done in a smooth and coordinated manner. It is useful to observe the patient's *handwriting;* alteration at times is indicative of subtle cerebellar dysfunction.

## Lower Extremities

### HEEL-KNEE TEST

With the patient in the supine position, the heel of one foot is placed on the opposite knee, a maneuver ordinarily carried out smoothly and accurately without tremor. The foot is then slid down the shin; again this is normally performed smoothly and evenly.

### PATTING TEST

The patient is requested to pat his foot quickly on the floor, in a manner similar to the hand patting test. As in the upper limb, this repetitive movement should be performed smoothly and regularly. Alternating abduction-adduction movement of the foot, using the heel as a fulcrum, may also be tested.

### FIGURE-OF-EIGHT TEST

While recumbent, the patient draws a figure-of-eight in the air with his great toe. This is normally done effectively and with dispatch.

## Trunk

The station and gait are both simply tested. The *station,* or stance, is tested by requesting the patient to stand in Romberg's position with the feet close together, first with the eyes open, then with the eyes closed. Additionally, he is asked to stand with one foot directly in front of the other (tandem Romberg). The coordination of the trunk is also assessed by testing the *gait.* The patient is asked to walk briskly with his eyes open and closed, and to turn quickly. He should also be requested to walk heel-to-toe in a straight line (tandem gait); this can be done normally without loss of balance. The presence of unsteadiness, lurching, or broadening of the base should be noted as indicators of abnormal performance. In addition, the patient may be asked to walk around a chair or to sit and rise quickly, thus demonstrating his ability to make rapid postural adjustments.

He may also be asked to rise from a reclining posture without a pillow and with the legs widely separated.

## SENSORY SYSTEM

A thorough examination of sensation includes investigation of superficial, or cutaneous, sensibility (touch, pain, heat, cold), deep sensibility (vibratory sense, position sense, deep pain), and a variety of discriminatory, so-called cortical or integrative, modalities. For accurate testing, the patient should be examined in a quiet room free of distraction by extraneous stimuli, and preferably when he is not fatigued. The examination itself should not be too lengthy, since the patient tires rapidly and responses as a result become increasingly inaccurate and unreliable. In a routine examination, sensation is ordinarily tested at the end of the examination when the patient is even more liable to fatigue. In view of such features, clearly contributing to an inaccurate clinical appraisal, this part of the examination should be repeated alone if alterations in sensation are found on the initial evaluation. As with other parts of the neurologic examination, it is best to use the patient as his own control, always comparing one side of the body with the other.

In evaluation of sensation, one must initially determine, in a qualitative sense, what elements of sensation are affected, if any. If alteration is found, an attempt should be made to assess the degree or severity of involvement and, finally, to map out regionally the distribution of the sensory impairment. A complete sensory loss is spoken of as anesthesia (touch) or analgesia (pain); partial sensory loss is referred to as hypesthesia or hypalgesia. In some instances, sensation is more keenly felt than normal, a state of affairs referred to as hyperesthesia, hyperalgesia, or hyperpathia. In determining the distribution of sensory change, it is essential to decide whether it corresponds to a peripheral nerve or spinal root distribution, whether it is a complete segmental sensory level as seen in transverse spinal cord lesions, a hemianesthesia, or a dissociated sensory syndrome, or whether it corresponds in type and distribution to a thalamic or hemispheric (cortical) locus (see Chapter 3).

### Touch

This sense is tested by means of a wisp of cotton, or by the examiner's finger, brought gingerly and lightly down on the skin. Tickling should be avoided, since this may represent subliminal pain.

### Pain

Pain is tested by means of a pin with which the patient is pricked over various parts of the skin surface. Normally the patient can readily distinguish between the point and head of the pin. When an area of impairment of pain sensibility is encountered, it should be mapped out by moving the stimulating pin from the impaired, or non-feeling, area to normal, asking the patient to indicate the line of demarcation or transition; the limits of the affected region may then be confirmed by moving the pin in the opposite direction (i.e., from feeling to non-feeling). When dealing with patients with cerebral lesions, it is also important to examine for sensory "extinction" or "inattention." This may be done by stimulating simultaneously opposite sides of the body in a symmetrical manner, determining whether pinprick or touch is obliterated on one side while still appreciated on the other; this has validity, it should be pointed out, only if individual stimuli are normally appreciated on either side alone.

## Heat and Cold

These modalities are commonly tested by utilizing test tubes containing hot water and cracked ice. Such extremes of temperature suffice for routine neurologic examination. Evaluation of these thermal modalities may be very helpful in refining the extent of the sensory defect originally discovered when testing for pain appreciation.

## Vibration Sense

This sense is examined by placing a vibrating C-128 tuning fork on various bony surfaces, in particular the wrist, elbow, ankle, and shin. The examiner interrupts the vibration as he desires and the patient is asked to state when the vibration ceases. In doubtful instances, this test may be quantitated, albeit crudely: the vibration of a C-128 fork is ordinarily felt on the back of the hand for 15 to 20 seconds in normal individuals, and over the tibia for 7 to 10 seconds, especially in the young. In patients over 50 years of age, vibratory sense is often impaired in the lower extremities.

## Position Sense

The thumb and great toe are grasped from the sides and gently moved; the patient is asked to state whether the digit is pointing up or down. Recognition of the initiation of movement may also be sought. Since clues as to the position of the digit may be derived from differential pressures perceived on the dorsal and volar (or plantar) surfaces, these should be avoided for the sake of accuracy.

## Two-Point Discrimination

A calibrated compass is utilized for this test. The patient is asked to indicate whether he feels one or two compass points over various points of the body. This test is perhaps most useful in disorders of the sensory cortex, but impairment may be found with lesions at lower levels. The normal threshold, or minimal recognizable separation, is 4 to 5 mm at the fingertips, much greater elsewhere.

## Stereognosis

The patient is asked, with the eyes closed, to identify the size, shape, and identity of common objects placed in the hand. Marbles, small cubes, coins, and safety pins are among the objects utilized for this purpose. Recognition of the nature of such objects is dependent initially on the integrity of tactile and proprioceptive sensation; if either of these modalities is impaired, the patient will be unable to identify objects held in the hand and may therefore present a spurious impression of astereognosis.

## Graphesthesia

Normal individuals can recognize numbers or letters traced on the skin with a blunt object. The palmar surface of the hand is generally used for this purpose, and the patient is asked to identify the number or letter so drawn.

## Tactile Localization

The patient is requested to indicate accurately, with his forefinger, a spot touched by the examiner with the eyes closed. Normally, such sensory localization is remarkably accurate over the fingers and hands, and relatively less precise more proximally.

## Texture and Weight Differentiation

Finally, differences in *texture* and *weight* of objects may be tested by asking the patient to identify various fabrics and materials in terms of texture and to determine the difference in weight of standardized blocks.

# EXAMINATION OF THE INFANT AND CHILD

The manner of examination suitable for older children and adults is not appropriate for the very young. Alternate modes of evaluation of the nervous system are necessary in light of the restrictions engendered by the patient's age. While a detailed description of the neurologic examination in the newborn, infant, and child is beyond the scope of this manual, it is appropriate here to indicate the general areas of interest to which attention must be directed in evaluating the neurologic status of these individuals. At the outset, it should be stressed that the newborn must be able to breathe on his own, to maintain his body temperature, and to feed, all functions essential in making the transition from an intrauterine to an extrauterine environment. Dysfunction in these spheres, along with poor response to stimulation, indicates significant neurologic difficulty requiring further investigation and care.

**HEAD CIRCUMFERENCE.** Undue alteration in head size may provide an early clue to the presence of intracranial disease. Head circumference must therefore be monitored periodically during infancy. Bear in mind that the average circumference of the head at birth is 34 cm, at one year 46 cm, and in adult life 54 cm in women, 56 cm in men. The state of the sutures and of the fontanels must also be assessed on a regular basis.

**COGNITIVE/ADAPTIVE BEHAVIOR.** Certain developmental milestones provide useful information regarding the acquisition of cognitive function; in fact, one may look upon the developmental examination in the infant as equivalent to examination of the mental status in the adult. Among the more useful parameters to be judged are such *fine motor skills* as the ability to transfer objects from hand to hand, generally present at 28 weeks; poking with the index finger, present by 40 weeks; the ability to build a tower of two blocks, appearing by 15 months; and the development of scribbling, usually by 18 months.

**GROSS MOTOR SKILLS.** In addition to fine skills, gross motor skills must also be evaluated. Pertinent landmarks include the ability to hold the head up to 90° when prone (i.e, achievement of head control), by 16 weeks; facility in rolling over from prone to supine, generally by 24 weeks; ability to sit up, ordinarily appearing at 6 to 9 months; creeping, generally at 9 to 10 months; standing alone, at 10 months; and walking, usually by 12 to 15 months.

**LANGUAGE.** The acquisition of language skills may also be assessed, at least indirectly. Thus, by 12 weeks cooing is noted, and by 28 weeks the normal infant is utilizing recurrent vowel sounds. The ability to use words is ordinarily manifest by 12 months, with a reasonable number of words available by 18 months; at this age, the infant can ordinarily identify pictures. At 24 months, the use of phrases and short sentences is evident, and by 36 months, at most, longer sentences appear.

**SPECIAL SENSES.** As regards the special senses, it should be recognized that the normal infant blinks to bright light at birth and is capable of following a light or other objects in the environment fully by 12 weeks of age. The normal infant will similarly blink to a loud sound at birth. By 12 to 16 weeks an infant can localize sounds, as evidenced, for example, by his turning the head to the source of noise.

**SOCIAL DEVELOPMENT.** Finally, personal and social development is appraised. Spontaneous smiling is normally observed at 8 weeks with responsive smiling appearing by 20 weeks. Effective social relationships are ordinarily well established by 5 months of age. Toilet training is normally accomplished by 2 to 3 years.

The above is clearly not intended as a detailed description of normal development, or its evaluation. These phenomena are simply exemplary of the more important modes of assessment of development applicable to infants and young children, and which provide at least indirectly required information as to the functioning of the nervous system. Clearly, other parameters must also be utilized, for example, investigation of the muscle stretch reflexes and at least crude appraisal of the ability to respond to certain forms of sensory stimulation. The neurologic evaluation of the very young individual is therefore substantially different from that of the adult; it is not, however, beyond the reach of the thoughtful practicing physician.

## BIBLIOGRAPHY


Cogan, D.G.: *Neurology of the Ocular Muscles.* ed. 2. Charles C Thomas, Springfield, Ill., 1963.

DeJong, R., and Magee, K.: *The Neurologic Examination.* ed. 4. Harper & Row, Hagerstown, 1979.

Medical Research Council: *Aids to the Investigation of Peripheral Nerve Injuries.* (Revised ed. 2, 1943.) Her Majesty's Stationery Office, London, reprinted 1967.

Paine, R. S., and Oppe, T. E.: *Neurological Examination of Children.* Lavenham Press, Ltd., Lavenham, Suffolk, 1966, reprinted 1971.

Strub, R. L., and Black, F. W.: *The Mental Status Examination in Neurology.* F. A. Davis, Philadelphia, 1977.

VanAllen, M. W., and Rodnitzky, R. L.: *Pictorial Manual of Neurologic Tests.* ed. 2. Year Book Medical Publishers, Inc., Chicago, 1981.

# 2

# INTERPRETATION OF NEUROLOGIC SYMPTOMS AND SIGNS

An exhaustive survey of the meaning of neurologic symptoms and signs would lead far afield. Nonetheless, some consideration of this aspect of the neurologic examination is essential here, since the attainment of a logical and accurate clinical diagnosis begins with the recognition of abnormal signs, followed by their proper analysis and appreciation of their functional significance. The more common abnormalities that may be encountered in a neurologic examination, therefore, merit description at this juncture.

## CONSCIOUSNESS

When a patient exhibits alteration in the state of awareness, an effort should be made to grade the changes in terms of severity or depth; this may be of considerable importance in judging the course of the patient's illness and, thus, of substantial import prognostically. The term *lethargy* indicates a state of drowsiness or inattention, with the patient dropping off to sleep frequently, although he is rousable to command. When stimulated, the patient's cooperation can ordinarily be enlisted, at least for a short time, but the attention span is abbreviated and he will again drop off to sleep. Responses may be delayed or incomplete, and little spontaneity of movement or thought is observed. In *stupor* the degree of physical and mental activity is minimal. The patient can be roused only with great difficulty and responds inadequately to events about him. Cooperation with the examination is slight. Periorbital reflex release and forced grasping may be encountered. A loss of the ability to respond to verbal stimuli with preservation of at least some arousal with painful stimuli is found in the state of *semi-coma*. Little movement is seen with the exception of decorticate or decerebrate posturing, which may appear either spontaneously or in response to noxious stimulation. Purposeful movements are fragmentary at best. Eye movements are often wandering or disconjugate. A decrease in reflex activity may be encountered; the plantar responses are often extensor. In *coma* there is no consistent response to either auditory or painful stimuli. Virtually no movements are seen. Reflexes are lost, periodic or depressed respirations are common, and pupillary abnormalities are frequent.

Plum and Posner have stressed the regular chain of events that accompanies central, or transtentorial, herniation consequent to an expanding supratentorial mass lesion. As a result of such a pattern of herniation, there is downward displacement and distortion of the brainstem. The resultant ischemia advances down the brainstem in a rostrocaudal sequence, producing serial functional levels of transection, evidenced by an orderly train of clinical abnormalities indicating subacute failure of first, diencephalic, then midbrain, pontine, and eventually medullary function. The clinical features of the stages so defined are summarized in Table 2-1. Two additional points should be made: (1) At the diencephalic stage, the process is potentially reversible. If relief is provided promptly, the prognosis is usually good for neurologic recovery. Once signs of midbrain dysfunction appear, however, the prognosis becomes much poorer, since at this stage ischemia has presumably already proceeded to irreversible changes with frank brainstem necrosis, particularly in the paramedian structures. (2) In uncal herniation with lateral brainstem compression, the stage of diencephalic dysfunction is commonly by-passed, and the patient rapidly develops features of midbrain abnormality. Thereafter, progression follows much the same pattern as noted in the individual with central, transtentorial herniation. Typically, signs of oculomotor nerve compression, particularly pupillary changes, appear early. The entire course of deterioration tends to be acute in uncal herniation, in contrast to the subacute evolution typical of transtentorial herniation.

Central to a discussion of depression of awareness is a consideration of so-called *irreversible coma (brain death, coma depassé)*. In this state, caused by either primary intracranial disease such as severe head injury or secondary to extracranial disorders, loss of cerebral autoregulation and total vasoparesis with failure of systemic vasopressor mechanisms lead to complete intracranial circulatory arrest. Severe and extensive necrosis of cerebral tissue results, such that *all* meaningful cerebral activity, including the ability to maintain respiratory and cardiovascular functions, is abolished. This is associated with a flat (i.e., isoelectric) electroencephalogram and with failure of filling of the intracranial vessels with attempted cerebral angiography. Even with the most intensive supportive therapeutic

**TABLE 2-1.** Stages in rostrocaudal deterioration with central (transtentorial) herniation (After Plum, F., and Posner, J. B.)

| STAGE | CONSCIOUSNESS | PUPILS | EYE MOVEMENTS | OCULO-VESTIBULAR RESPONSES | RESPIRATION | MOTOR FUNCTION | OTHER |
|---|---|---|---|---|---|---|---|
| Diencephalic | Somnolence, stupor, coma | Small, slightly reactive | Roving, conjugate | Abnormal calorics; doll's head responses brisk | Sighing; Cheyne-Stokes | Generalized hypertonicity; bilateral pyramidal tract signs; decorticate posturing | |
| Midbrain-Upper Pontine | Coma | Mid-size, fixed | Dysconjugate | Difficult to elicit | Central neurogenic hyperventilation | Bilateral decerebrate posturing | Hyperthermia/ Hypothermia; occasionally diabetes insipidus |
| Lower Pontine-Upper Medullary | Coma | Mid-size, fixed | Absent | Absent | Tachypnea | Generalized flaccidity; bilateral extensor plantars; minimal flexion withdrawal | |
| Medullary (Terminal) | Coma | Dilated, fixed | Absent | Absent | Ataxic; periodic; apnea | Flaccidity | Pulse variable, peripheral vascular collapse. |

efforts, circulatory failure is inevitable: cardiac arrest ordinarily ensues within 3 to 5 days of onset in adults, perhaps somewhat longer in children. Appreciation of this state of brain death has assumed major importance in recent years, parallelling broadened interest in, and successful utilization of, organ transplantation techniques made possible in turn by the development of aggressive and increasingly effective supportive medical therapy for the critically ill. The ethical and medicolegal ramifications are substantial. There are as yet, however, no universally accepted criteria applicable to such putative brain death cases. Rigorously excluded in the consideration of brain death, but at times capable of mimicking this state of irreversible coma, are instances of severe drug intoxication and of profound hypothermia.

Several clinical states must be clearly distinguished from instances of irreversible coma. In *akinetic mutism,* or *coma vigil,* the patient exhibits no voluntary movements, demonstrates no emotional expression, and remains mute. However, the patient frequently appears aware, exhibits definite sleep-waking cycles, will open the eyes, and seems able to fix on, and follow, events in the environment. Primitive functions such as sucking, chewing, and swallowing may be preserved and oculocephalic responses are intact. The patient is not necessarily totally akinetic; in response to very painful stimuli, fragmentary and ineffective withdrawal may be seen. This state is a consequence of lesions in the vicinity of the third ventricle, or of bilateral lesions in the thalamus, basal ganglia, midbrain, or cingulate gyrus. Such patients, it should be emphasized, are capable of maintaining circulatory and respiratory functions unassisted. In the *apallic state,* the patient exhibits a loss of all higher function, tending to exhibit a chronic decorticate posture with little or no spontaneous movements. He appears awake, but without evidence of emotional reactions or of ocular fixation or pursuit in response to environmental events. In this state, which results from diffuse and severe gray and/or white matter disease involving the cerebral hemispheres, brainstem functions are preserved, and primitive perioral and forced grasping reflexes are easily elicited. Finally, the term *parasomnia* refers to a state of persistent pathologic sleep following trauma to the upper brainstem. The designation *persistent vegetative state,* or vegetative survival, is sometimes applied to all these clinical states in an indiscriminate manner.

The so-called *locked-in syndrome* must be sharply distinguished from these states of altered awareness. In this disorder, a patient is rendered mute and virtually immobile by virtue of bilateral lesions, almost always in the basis pontis. In such individuals, awareness is commonly intact, and the problem is essentially one of inability to respond to environmental stimuli by virtue of a severe paralysis of all the limbs, and of bulbar function as well. The patient is thus mute and tetraplegic but is fully alert, since the reticular activating system and hemispheres are spared. With patience, he can learn to communicate effectively by utilizing an eye-blink code—eye closure is curiously preserved as virtually the only volitional movement available. This is thus a problem of immobility and incapacity to communicate rather than of impairment of consciousness as such.

*Confusion* is a state characterized by an inability to think with ordinary clarity and coherence; it is generally associated with a lack of spontaneous speech and some degree of lethargy. Disorientation and perceptual misinterpretations and distortions are common. When psychomotor and autonomic overactivity are added to the syndrome of confusion, the term *delirium* is employed; a *beclouded delirium* is a delirious state added to an antecedent dementia.

## MENTATION

Turning now to testing of *mentation* (i.e, of cognitive function and of memory), the general pattern of response of the patient must be analyzed carefully at the outset. Slow, hesitant replies may be of great significance, presuming that they are not normal for the person in question. Such slowness, or *bradyphrenia,* which may be looked upon as an expression of delay in the processing of symbolic bits of information, is commonly observed in the individual with organic intellectual impairment, but may also be found in the patient with aphasia. It should not be confused with the slow, hesitant verbalizations of the patient with parkinsonism or other dysarthric disorders.

*Dementia* (organic mental syndrome, chronic brain syndrome) appears in a number of circumstances. It is characterized by loss or impairment of memory, especially for events of the recent past; a shortened attention span, often associated with ease of distractability and difficulty in concentration; reduction in learning capacity; impairment in the ability to comprehend abstract concepts and to synthesize ideas; and difficulty with simple arithmetic problems. Changes in judgment, personality, mood, and affect often accompany the cognitive defect. Such a clinical constellation may be manifest in any condition in which there is diffuse or extensive destruction of the cerebral cortex or underlying white matter. It must be emphasized that in general the observation of dementia does not *per se* indicate a specific, isolated site within the cerebrum whose destruction results in the appearance of this symptom complex. Lesions responsible for such global intellectual impairment may be found in either the gray or white matter, or both, and in either cerebral hemisphere. No specific lobe or major subdivision thereof can be implicated exclusively, and at times the responsible lesion actually appears to be in the central gray structures rather than more superficially in the hemispheres themselves. Ancillary localizing neurologic signs, such as visual field abnormalities or hemiparesis, must therefore be sought to permit precise clinical localization in the demented patient. There are, however, certain varieties of mental dysfunction that are of greater anatomic specificity and that warrant further description here.

The term *amnestic dementia* is applied to a syndrome characterized by a profound disorder of memory, especially for memories of the recent past (and suggesting an inability to form or store new memories), with largely intact memory for the more remote past and relative preservation of other cognitive functions. This is the central defect in Korsakoff's psychosis and appears to reflect bilateral lesions in the mammillary bodies and/or dorsal thalamus. It may also be observed in patients with bilateral lesions involving the mesial (hippocampal) structures of the temporal lobes, or, at times, the fornix. Finally, it may be encountered with tumors of the third ventricle or hypothalamus, which compress or destroy the pillars of the fornix, the mammillary bodies, or the mammillothalamic tract. Particularly in the face of mesial temporal lesions, as in herpes simplex encephalitis or occlusive vascular disease affecting the posterior cerebral arteries, the rubric *limbic dementia* is sometimes applied; patients so designated evidence, in addition to a defect in memory, behavioral and affective changes and commonly dysphasia or cortical blindness. The term *thalamic dementia* refers to those rare cases of bilateral destructive thalamic lesions that demonstrate clinically memory impairment along with defective attention and vigilance. Finally, an isolated impairment in the ability to calculate (acalculia), with preservation of other intellectual functions, is found in the *Gerstmann syndrome,* which ordinarily appears as a consequence of a destructive lesion in the angular and/or supermarginal gyri of the dominant cerebral hemisphere (see below).

The *personality* changes found in organic brain disease are not specifically indicative of frontal lobe disease, as is often thought, but do occur with disorders of this area particularly frequently. The fundamental feature is a change in the normal mode of reaction of the affected person. Mistakes in judgment, loss of niceties of social interaction, coarse or overtly antisocial behavior, sexual excesses and indiscretions, and other nonspecific forms of abnormal reaction are encountered. The particular alteration varies widely from patient to patient, but of basic importance is a change from the premorbid personality structure. At times one observes an intensification of previous personality traits. Mood disturbances and, in particular, rapid mood swings also occur with organic brain disease. These too have no localizing significance and are usually associated with a diffuse lesion. Emotional lability characterized by loss of control and easy crying and laughing without adequate stimulus may be encountered in patients with multiple sclerosis or in demented individuals and is typically observed in patients suffering from bilateral pyramidal tract disease with *pseudobulbar palsy.* Inappropriate laughter may also occur as part of a seizure in so-called *gelastic epilepsy,* a form of temporal lobe epilepsy. A curious syndrome of facetiousness with senseless jokes and puns, referred to as *witzelsucht,* may also be found in patients with disease of the cerebrum. Impulsive, even aggressive, behavior is found at times in postencephalitic states and in epileptics, especially those with psychomotor seizures, a behavioral alteration sometimes referred to as a *dyscontrol syndrome.* Euphoria is occasionally found in patients with multiple sclerosis, although probably less often than either depression or dementia; when present, it appears to reflect a lack of insight as a result of loss of the patient's ability to assess, evaluate, and appreciate his own deficit. Apathy may appear in the course of many organic disorders. Finally, a depressive reaction may develop with a variety of intrinsic diseases of the brain, perhaps most commonly as a simple reactive phenomenon.

Among the higher skilled or integrative acts that may be disturbed in patients with organic disease of the brain is *language.* This may be manifested by aphasia, that is, a disorder of symbolic language, or by dysarthria, a term referring merely to disturbance in enunciation. *Aphasia* (see Chapter 3), or dysphasia, is characterized by difficulty in the formulation, expression, integration, or comprehension of language. It may be evidenced simply by a readily identifiable inability to find words, a defect of which the patient is ordinarily aware and capable of describing; or by a severe and disabling defect in expression, with considerable loss of words; or by a gross defect in understanding; or by a combination of these. Other defects in the use of symbolic language, such as an inability to read (dyslexia, alexia) and to write (dysgraphia, agraphia), generally accompany disorders of spoken language.

The term *dysarthria,* on the other hand, refers to impairment in the rate, rhythm, quality, and intonation of the voice and to defective modulation (prosody) and articulation of sounds. Dysarthria is due to a defect in the muscular control of the peripheral speech apparatus, but the central symbolic aspect of language is preserved. It is often tested by requesting the patient to repeat certain test phrases, such as "Massachusetts artillery," "particular statistics," "truly rural," "Irish constabulary," or "round the rugged rock the ragged rascal ran." Dysarthria may result from lesions of either the central or the peripheral nervous system. A variety of forms can be identified whose recognition may yield important information as to the location and nature of the underlying disease process. For example, in instances of pseudobulbar palsy with bilateral corticospinal and corticobulbar disease, a *spastic dysarthria* is encountered, which is characterized by imprecision of consonants, monotony of pitch, and irregular loudness, along with a strained, almost strangled quality. The voice may be nasal; nasality is much more prominent in the *flaccid dysarthria* of bulbar palsy and reflects weakness of the palatal, pharyngeal, and perhaps lingual muscles. The speech under these circumstances is quite muffled, often with a slow and sibilant quality, and defective articulation of consonants is found. In a disease such as amyotrophic lateral sclerosis, features of both bulbar and pseudobulbar speech are identifiable; inappropriate silences and gaps between words and prolongation of phonemes are additionally encountered. In cerebellar disease, in contrast, an *ataxic dysarthria* appears, which is considered a reflection of dysynergia of the speech apparatus. An irregular pattern of articulation with a tendency to telescope single or sequential syllables is typical, and a thickened quality is characteristic. A *scanning* speech may be observed in these patients, characterized by excessive stress on parts of speech that are normally unstressed; slowing of speech and the occurrence of unduly long intervals between phonemes or words, or both, are also found. In parkinsonism a dysarthric defect sometimes referred to as *hypokinetic dysarthria* is encountered. The speech is muffled and monotonous in both pitch and loudness; imprecision of articulation, harshness or sibilance, variability in rate, and inappropriate silences may be noted. During the course of conversation, the speech tends to fade away into an unintelligible murmur. Patients with chorea and dystonia exhibit excessive variations in loudness and in rate of speech, a disorder sometimes called *hyperkinetic dysarthria.* In a variety of other conditions, such as general paresis, a simple slurring dysarthria may be found. Even so simple a disorder as a peripheral facial palsy (Bell's palsy) may be accompanied by a thickening and distortion of speech.

The *body scheme,* or image, is an unconscious construct (gestalt) comprising one's image of the relationship of parts of the body to each other, of one side of the body to the other, and of the body as a whole to surrounding, extracorporeal space. It appears to develop during infancy and childhood on the basis of tactile, proprioceptive, and visual experiences. Disorders of the body scheme may appear with organic disease of the brain and are particularly common with lesions involving the minor (nondominant) parietal lobe. *Unilateral neglect* (inattention) most frequently affects the left side and may be motor, sensory, or mixed. An example is *dressing apraxia,* in which the patient neglects to dress the left side while clothing himself, but the term neglect is in fact used for any disregard of the left side during voluntary activity. Sensory neglect is brought out by utilizing double simultaneous stimulation (tactile, painful, visual, or auditory); although capable of appreciating such modalities when tested on either side alone, the patient ignores them on the affected side when both sides are tested at the same time. That such a pattern of neglect may extend to extracorporeal space is well demonstrated by defects in drawing symmetrical forms, such as the face of a clock or a flower, or in design copying.

In a more striking vein, the patient may also be unaware of, or actively deny, the presence of a hemiparesis or hemiplegia, ordinarily involving the left side; this defect is called *anosognosia* (it should be noted that this term is sometimes used in a much broader sense to indicate denial of any form of somatic illness; when so used, it lacks the relatively precise anatomic connotation described here). An occasional patient may actually deny the existence of the left side of the body, a state of affairs referred to as *hemisomatotopagnosia* (or amorphosynthesis or hemidepersonalization). In general, disorders of the body scheme are accompanied by alteration of sensation, most importantly of proprioception, and by varying degrees of mental confusion. Abruptly evolving lesions are most likely to be associated with the appearance of these deficits; as a result, defects of this sort are usually found in patients with cerebrovascular disease. The fact that body scheme disorders are more consistently encountered in patients with nondominant rather than dominant hemisphere lesions may simply reflect the fact that vascular accidents involving the dominant hemisphere tend to be associated with aphasia, which makes it difficult or impossible to communicate with the patient sufficiently to elicit these rather subtle abnormalities.

Yet another defect in the body scheme, not necessarily associated with mental or sensory changes, is right-left disorientation, which is commonly associated with finger agnosia, dysgraphia, and acalculia in the Gerstmann syndrome. This is observed most frequently with lesions involving the dominant parietotemporal region, and is thus in distinct contrast to the deficits described hitherto. Additionally, it is recognized that very severe disorders of the body scheme may appear in a variety of other disorders that are not related to focal structural alteration of the brain *per se,* for example, acute psychosis and drug intoxication. In these instances, such symptoms are usually not lateralizing in quality and would appear to reflect generalized neuronal dysfunction. They are not likely to be confused with the more specific body scheme disorders resulting from focal brain disease.

## CRANIAL NERVES

### Olfactory (I)

*Anosmia,* or complete loss of smell, is found most commonly as a result of local disease involving the olfactory bulb, nerve, and tract. It is only rarely noted with lesions involving the more central olfactory connections and is frequently overlooked by the patient, who may be totally unaware of such a complete loss of smell. Anosmia occurs with meningiomas involving the olfactory groove, or with trauma affecting the ethmoid plate, and is associated with laceration of the base of the frontal lobe. Under such circumstances leakage of spinal fluid through the nose may also be noted. A reduced sense of smell is also often encountered in normal individuals (e.g., as a result of nasal obstruction or acute upper respiratory infection) and is commonly of little clinical importance. Impairment of the sense of smell (hyposmia), and generally of taste as well (hypogeusia), accompanied by distorted perceptions involving these sensory modalities, commonly follows a viral respiratory illness; a deficiency of zinc has been implicated in its pathogenesis. Repugnant smells occur as olfactory hallucinations, at times associated with hallucinations of taste, as part of so-called uncinate fits and are generally taken to indicate a lesion (epileptogenic focus) involving the anterior and mesial portion of the temporal lobe; lip smacking and chewing movements may accompany these hallucinatory experiences.

## Optic (II)

Diseases of the optic nerve are characterized by (1) disturbance or loss of visual acuity, commonly associated with defective color vision, (2) pupillary abnormalities, (3) visual field defects, and (4) changes in the fundus oculi. The nerve may be involved primarily by trauma and by a host of inflammatory and compressive lesions anywhere between the retina and the optic chiasm. Such affections are commonly associated with the appearance of primary optic atrophy. The optic nerve also may be involved secondarily, as in the process of progressive organization and gliosis leading to the appearance of secondary or consecutive optic atrophy in patients with increased intracranial pressure and papilledema.

### VISUAL LOSS

Disease of the optic nerve is frequently associated with partial or complete loss of vision (amblyopia). In the case of tumors that compress or infiltrate the optic nerves this impairment is usually slowly progressive, whereas in other disorders, such as retrobulbar neuritis or papillitis, ischemic optic neuritis, or nutritional amblyopia, the visual loss may be acute or subacute in presentation. In papilledema caused by increased intracranial pressure, the visual acuity is ordinarily preserved, but may deteriorate subsequently as secondary ("consecutive") optic atrophy ensues. When the visual acuity falls as a result of disease of the optic nerve, color vision is usually impaired as well, not unexpectedly in view of the fact that both central and color vision are mediated by the macular cones. A loss of image brightness or intensity may appear as an early subtle manifestation of such an anteriorly placed lesion.

A special form of visual impairment is *night blindness,* that is, impairment of visual acuity when the ambient illumination is low. This is found primarily with disease of the retina, rather than of the optic nerve, and is encountered typically in vitamin A deficiency states, which in turn reflect a deficiency of rhodopsin (visual purple). Night blindness is also encountered in the earlier phases of retinitis pigmentosa, a commonly familial degenerative disorder involving particularly the rod cells of the retina. Finally, *transient obscurations* of vision may be encountered in a variety of circumstances, including the so-called hydrocephalic crises of increased intracranial pressure, episodes of transient cerebrovascular insufficiency in patients with carotid artery stenosis (referred to here as *amaurosis fugax*), and migraine.

### PUPILLARY CHANGES

Pupillary abnormalities are common in the face of optic nerve disease and reflect interruption of the afferent portion of the light reflex arc. With acute affections of the optic nerve, the pupil is often dilated to at least some extent. The involved pupil fails to react to direct light, but the consensual response is preserved. Very often, a seemingly paradoxical dilatation of the pupil may be observed with the swinging-light test (Marcus-Gunn deafferented pupil). Other pupillary changes are described below.

## VISUAL FIELD DEFECTS

Defects in the visual field are found in virtually all optic nerve afflictions and, in fact, in a variety of disorders involving all portions of the visual conducting apparatus from the retina to the calcarine cortex. Precise mapping of the visual field abnormality in any given patient is often of great assistance in localizing lesions accurately. Thus, highly characteristic abnormalities of the visual fields are found in patients with disease of the *retina* itself. With local retinal disease, such as a patch of chorioretinitis or a retinal tear, arc-shaped sector defects are characteristic. In glaucoma, step-like fiber bundle scotomata appear. With a focal lesion involving the macula itself, a central scotoma is typical. In contrast, with diffuse disorders of the more peripheral portions of the retina, such as retinitis pigmentosa, a generalized constriction of the field may occur. At times, it should be pointed out, such a peripheral constriction must be distinguished from so-called tubular ("gun barrel") vision as encountered in the hysteric. This may be effected most simply by doubling the distance of the patient from the tangent screen; in organic retinal disease, the seeing portion of the field will enlarge in a ratio determined by the square of the distance from the screen, in accordance with basic physical principles, whereas in hysteria the size of the field remains unchanged.

When the *optic nerve* is involved in its course from the retina to the

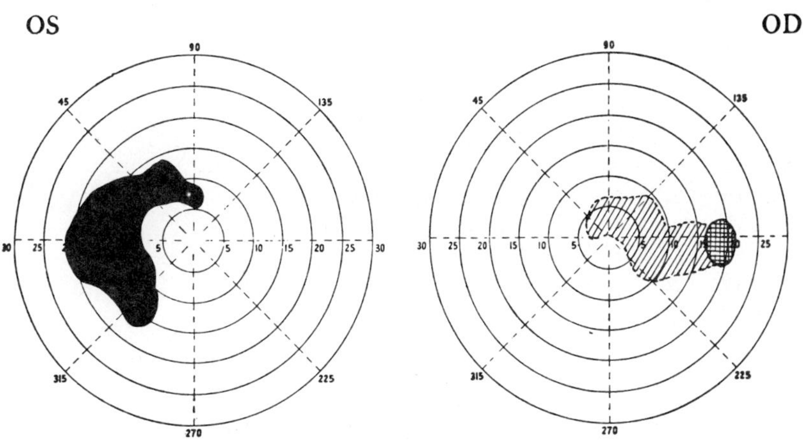


**FIGURE 2-1.** Absolute paracentral scotoma in left eye and relative central-paracentral scotoma in right eye in a patient with multiple sclerosis.

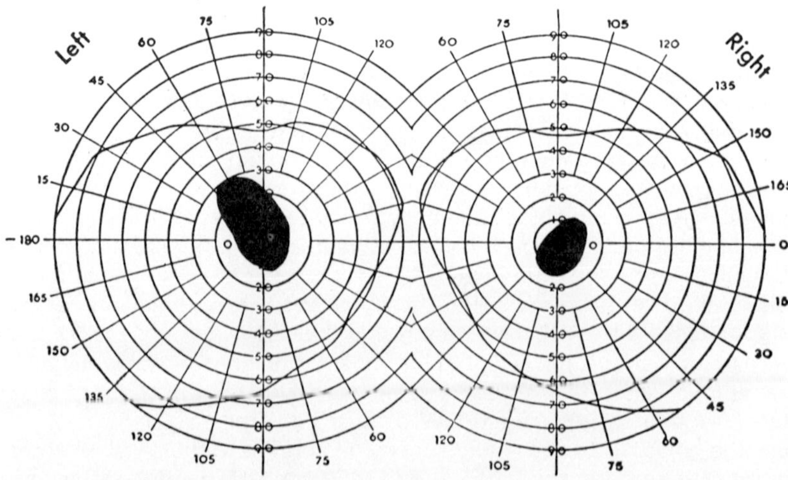


**FIGURE 2-2.** Central scotomas in a case of multiple sclerosis, with greatly reduced central vision.

optic chiasm, the visual field defect is usually a *scotoma,* which may be central, paracentral, or cecocentral (i.e., extending laterally to include the blind spot), depending upon the extent of nerve damage (Figs. 2-1 and 2-2). With central scotomatous defects, which imply affection of the macular fibers, there is always loss of visual acuity. Characteristically, the field defect of an optic nerve lesion is monocular. At times, especially with an infiltrating tumor posteriorly placed in the optic nerve, a so-called *junctional syndrome* appears, with a bilateral field defect indicating extension of the lesion back into the more anterior portion of the chiasm. Sector defects may be seen with optic nerve lesions. On occasion, an upper or lower field may be selectively obliterated; such defects, called *altitudinal,* are seen, for example, with subfrontal tumors compressing the optic nerve from above.

In disorders involving the optic chiasm, tract, or radiation, the field defect is *hemianopic,* involving portions of the field of both eyes, in contrast to the monocular distribution characteristic of the more anterior optic nerve lesions. Such hemianopic defects may be *congruous* or *incongruous:* in an incongruous field defect one field is affected much more than the other, whereas in a congruous defect they are equally affected. Such hemianopias may be bitemporal, binasal, or homonomous.

**BITEMPORAL HEMIANOPSIA.** This type of hemianopsia is characterized by the loss of both temporal fields of vision. The visual field defect in bitemporal hemianopsia is often through the fixation point and thus involves central vision. It is due to compression or disease of the optic chiasm, particularly involving those fibers decussating within it that are derived from the nasal sides of the retinae. The presence of a bitemporal hemianopsia indicates a lesion above the sella turcica, in the majority of instances a primary pituitary tumor growing upward from the sella and expanding through the diaphragma sella to compress the chiasm from below (Fig. 2-3). This defect may also be due to lesions originating above the sella, such as craniopharyngioma, tuberculum sella meningioma, aneurysm, or arachnoiditis. Parasellar lesions may cause a bitemporal hemianopsia by virtue of medial extension that compresses the chiasm. In rare instances a bitemporal hemianopsia results from craniocerebral trauma with laceration of the optic chiasm, or from downward pressure by a dilated third ventricle in instances of internal hydrocephalus caused by posterior fossa tumor. It should be noted that the exact position of the optic chiasm *vis-à-vis* the sella turcica varies from individual to individual, an anatomic variation that may have some influence upon the precise nature of the field defect encountered with suprasellar mass lesions. At times, the chiasm sits above and somewhat anterior to the sella (prefixed chiasm), and at other times above and slightly behind (postfixed); instead of a pure bitemporal hemianopsia, mixed field abnormalities may appear as a result of such anatomic variations. Variations in blood supply to the chiasm may also play a role in determining the exact field defect resulting from a compressing lesion.

**BINASAL HEMIANOPSIA.** A loss of the nasal halves of the field of vision is characteristic of this variety of field cut; it is thus the exact opposite of a bitemporal hemianopsia. It is produced by lesions that com-

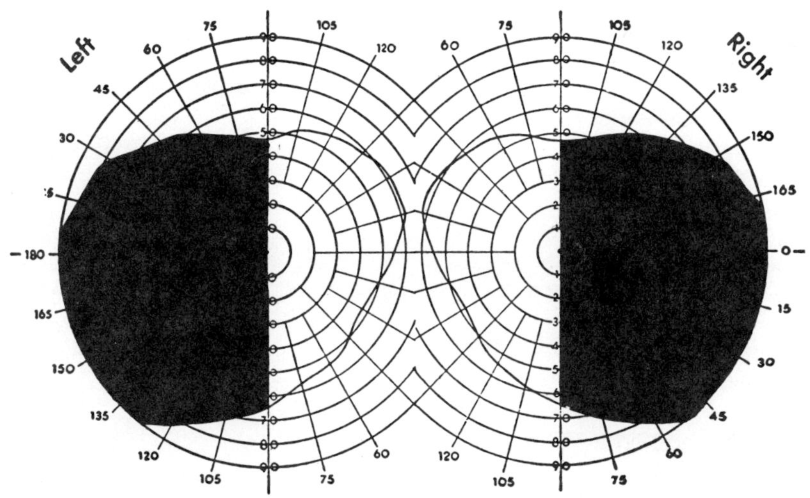


**FIGURE 2-3.** Bitemporal hemianopsia, in semidiagrammatic form, due to compression of the optic chiasm by a pituitary tumor.

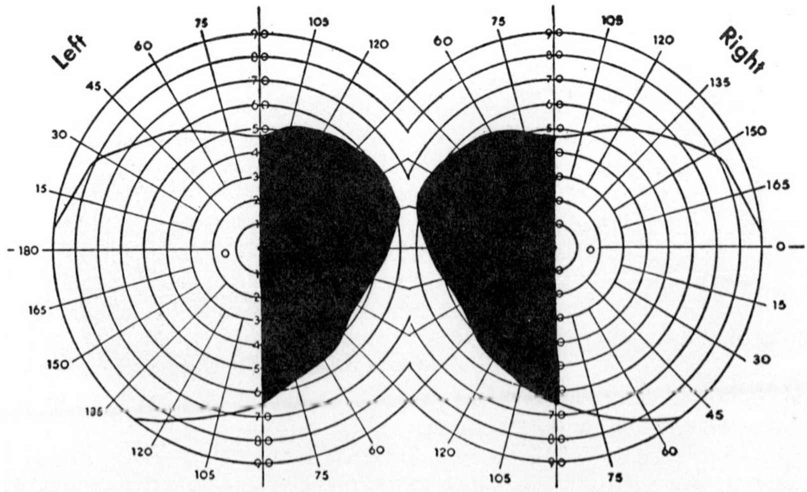


**FIGURE 2-4.** Binasal hemianopsia, a rare form of visual field defect, in this case caused by interruption of the fibers from the temporal sides of the retinae by compression from sclerosed internal carotid arteries.

press the optic chiasm from the side and compromise fibers originating in the temporal portions of each retina, and is most commonly encountered with fusiform atherosclerotic aneurysms of the internal carotid arteries (Fig. 2-4).

**HOMONYMOUS HEMIANOPSIA.** This is characterized by loss of the temporal field of one eye and the nasal field of the other (Fig. 2-5). The homonymous half fields are generally involved in their entirety; occasionally, a quadrantic defect (quadrantanopsia) appears. The field defect may spare or involve central vision. Homonymous hemianopsia results from disease of the optic tract or radiation from the optic chiasm to the termination of the visual pathways in the occipital lobe. Involvement of the optic tract itself (i.e., that portion of the visual conducting system between the chiasm and the lateral geniculate body) is most commonly due to tumor, aneurysm, or trauma. The optic radiations beyond the geniculate body in the temporal and occipital white matter may be involved by a variety of lesions, including softening, hemorrhage, tumor, abscess, and demyelinating disease. Homonymous hemianopsia caused by a tract lesion is generally accompanied by pupillary abnormalities, whereas these are not found when the lesion is posterior to the geniculate body.

Differences in the configuration of the visual fields have been used to define the precise localization of the lesions responsible, but these have only limited value. Thus, homonymous field defects through the fixation point are said to indicate temporal lobe lesions, since the fibers are closely

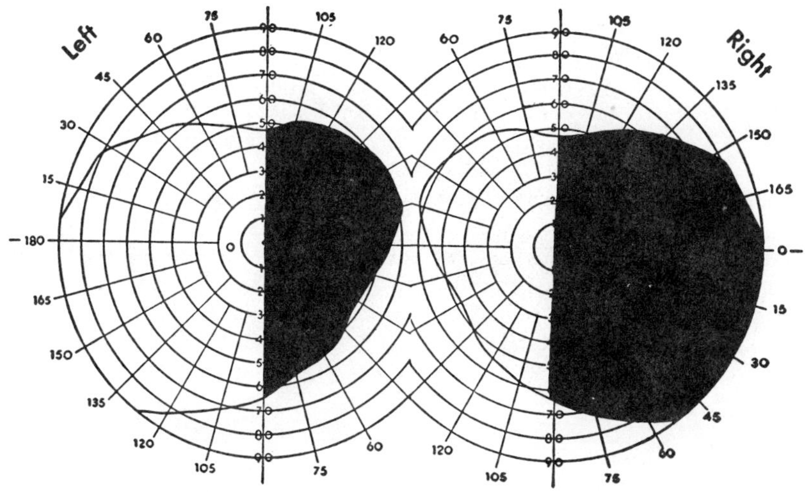


**FIGURE 2-5.** Homonymous hemianopsia (right) due to interruption of the visual pathways in the left temporal lobe in a case of brain tumor.

packed together here, while defects with sparing of the point of fixation are more likely to be due to occipital lesions. Though this is true to a limited degree it is not invariably the case. Involvement of central vision may occur in occipital lobe lesions, and sparing of central vision may occur with temporal lobe lesions. Faulty fixation on the part of the patient during field testing probably accounts for at least some of this uncertainty. It is usually asserted that a lesion of the optic tract can be differentiated from one involving the radiation by virtue of the fact that the

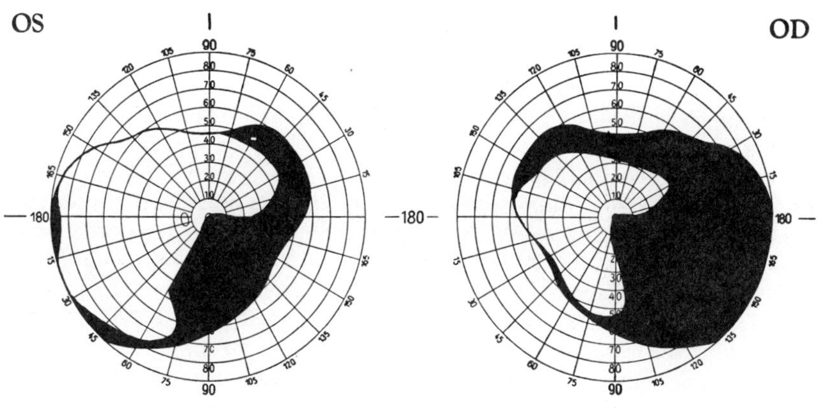


**FIGURE 2-6.** Incongruous right homonymous hemianopsia observed in a patient with a lesion involving the left optic tract.

field cut in the former tends to be incongruous (i.e., the field of one eye is affected more than the other) (Fig. 2-6), and in the latter congruous (i.e., identical in both eyes) (Fig. 2-7). Again, this is not a constant feature. In general, a search for accompanying focal neurologic signs may well prove more helpful in identifying the precise site of a lesion in these more posterior portions of the conducting system.

Under some circumstances only parts of the homonymous fields are affected. As indicated above, a quadrantic field defect, referred to as *quadrantanopsia,* involving either the upper or lower homonymous quadrants, may be seen. A superior or upper quadrantanopsia is likely to result from a temporal lobe lesion, such as a tumor expanding into the lower fibers of the optic radiation, whereas an inferior or lower quadrantanopsia

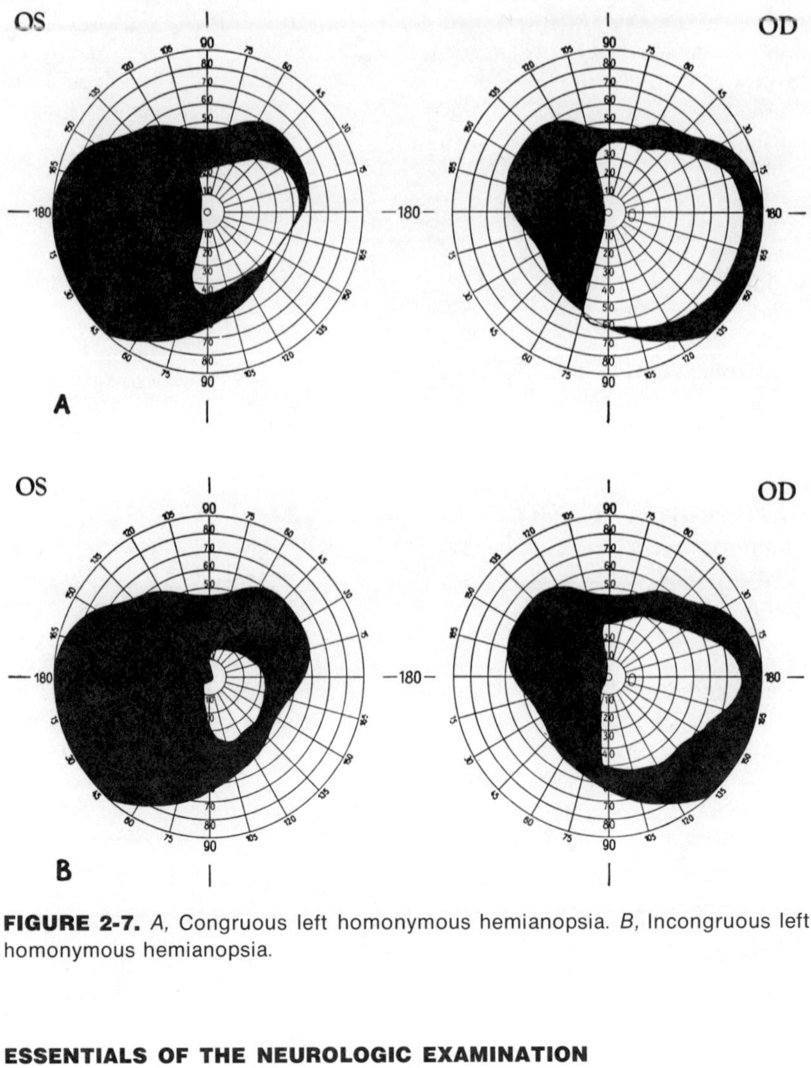


**FIGURE 2-7.** *A,* Congruous left homonymous hemianopsia. *B,* Incongruous left homonymous hemianopsia.

reflects involvement of the upper part of the radiation in or adjacent to the parietal lobe.

Under rare circumstances, a lesion of the optic radiation, usually a tumor, may produce a *crescentic* or hemicrescentic defect in the vision of one eye, without involvement of the homonymous field of the opposite eye. The defect is in the peripheral temporal field, representing the uniocular field of vision. Such field defects usually begin in the periphery and advance toward the center, frequently sparing central vision; they regress in reverse manner.

## OPTIC NERVE ABNORMALITIES

**PRIMARY OPTIC ATROPHY.** The most important neurologic conditions associated with primary optic atrophy include (1) mass lesions such as pituitary or suprasellar neoplasm, sphenoid ridge or olfactory groove meningiomas, and aneurysms; (2) inflammatory disorders, including tertiary syphilis (luetic optic atrophy); (3) demyelinating diseases, particularly multiple sclerosis; (4) heredodegenerative conditions such as Friedreich's ataxia and other spinocerebellar degenerations, Leber's hereditary optic atrophy, and primary retinal degenerations such as retinitis pigmentosa; (5) intoxication caused by such substances as arsenic, lead, quinine, and methyl alcohol; (6) other metabolic disorders such as hypoxia or pernicious anemia; (7) trauma; and (8) glaucoma, an often overlooked cause of optic atrophy.

**SECONDARY (CONSECUTIVE) OPTIC ATROPHY.** This condition develops in optic nerves that have been previously inflamed or edematous and in which organization and gliosis has occurred. It may follow optic neuritis, choked disc, or occlusive vascular disease.

**PAPILLEDEMA (CHOKED DISC, DISCEDEMA).** Papilledema, a noninflammatory edema of the optic nerve head, appears in the face of increased intracranial pressure, regardless of cause, and probably reflects venous congestion and interference with venous outflow. It is seen, for example, in instances of expanding intracranial lesions, such as brain tumor, epidural and subdural hematoma, or brain abscess; in chronic granulomatous meningitis with obstructive hydrocephalus; in acute infectious or metabolic encephalopathies of diverse causation associated with diffuse brain swelling; and in pseudotumor cerebri (so-called benign intracranial hypertension). Papilledema may also be found in situations in which the presence of heightened intracranial pressure is less convincing, such as polycythemia or in association with the Guillain-Barré syndrome. It is characterized by swelling and at times hyperemia of the optic nerve head, associated with dilatation and tortuosity of the retinal veins. The nerve head is elevated above the level of the retina; the edges of the nerve are first obscured, then completely obliterated. Changes appear first on the nasal aspect of the disc. The surrounding retina demonstrates no change initially, but edema subsequently spreads onto the retina; retinal folds may appear, hemorrhages and exudates develop, and a radiating macular star may be manifest. The elevation of the nerve head in choked disc may be measured by focusing the ophthalmoscope first on the retina at some distance from the disc, then on the edematous nerve head itself. The difference between the two readings represents the elevation of the choked disc as measured in diopters of swelling (1D, 2D, etc.). About 3D of swelling is equivalent to 1 mm of elevation of the nerve head itself. Because of varying degrees of accommodation on the part of the examiner, the measurement of disc elevation in diopters may be misleading and should not be considered precise.

The choked disc eventually becomes organized and replaced by glial tissue; the edema recedes and the nerve head becomes visible once again as gliosis proceeds. Secondary optic atrophy ultimately develops, and the nerve head appears grayish or grayish-white, with the edges indistinct in outline.

Some conditions mimic papilledema and must be carefully excluded from consideration. Both *drusen* (congenital refractile hyaline bodies) and *medullated* (myelinated) *nerve fibers* may lead to confusion in some patients, although they should be distinguished funduscopically with little difficulty. The term *pseudopapilledema* is sometimes applied to such misleading conditions. The swelling and hyperemia of the disc noted in acute optic neuritis or *papillitis* may on inspection also be confused with true papilledema. Ordinarily, loss of visual acuity and of color vision, along with a central scotoma, is found in instances of optic neuritis and serves to distinguish this condition from true papilledema, in which the visual acuity is generally normal and the visual fields abnormal only in terms of enlargement of the blind spot.

In addition to alterations in appearance of the optic nerve head itself, a number of other abnormalities that are encountered on funduscopic examination may prove to be of interest to the neurologist. These include the corpuscular pattern of pigmentary degeneration of the retina, as in retinitis pigmentosa; patches of chorioretinitis found in a number of disorders, such as toxoplasmosis and syphilis; macular degeneration; ischemic changes caused by occlusive disease involving the ophthalmic and/or retinal vessels; and subhyaloid hemorrhage in instances of subarachnoid hemorrhage. Also found are so-called Roth spots in patients with bacterial endocarditis with embolization; the cherry red spot in the macula in cases of Tay-Sachs disease; cholesterol-containing arterial plugs (Hollenhorst plaques) in cases of amaurosis fugax caused by intravascular microembolization; elevation of the entire central part of the retina, with a macular scar, in patients with loss of central vision and visual distortion in central serous retinitis; and many other abnormalities. The importance of an adequate ophthalmoscopic examination can thus hardly be overestimated.

## Oculomotor (III), Trochlear (IV), Abducens (VI)

Diseases of the ocular nerves produce disturbances of ocular motility (ocular palsy, ophthalmoplegia) and, in the case of the oculomotor nerve itself, pupillary alterations as well.

### PUPILS

Abnormalities of the pupils are commonly found in diseases involving the oculomotor nerve, but may of course appear with lesions involving other portions of the reflex pupillomotor mechanism, such as the optic nerve, as already discussed. The normal pupil is round, centrally placed, regular in outline, and equal in size to its fellow and responds promptly to light, both direct and indirect (consensual), and to accommodation. Unequal pupils *(anisocoria)* may be observed in otherwise entirely normal individuals. Unequal, irregular pupils that react slowly to light are found in neurosyphilis and occasionally in other conditions. A pupil may be said to be slow, or sluggish, in its reaction when it contracts slowly or imperfectly to direct light, and over a less than anticipated range. After contraction, such a pupil will ordinarily relax almost immediately. The *Argyll-Robertson pupil* is found typically in tabes dorsalis, less frequently in other forms of neurosyphilis. It has also been described in a number of other conditions, including encephalitis, multiple sclerosis, infiltrating tumors of the midbrain, and diabetes. Isolated loss of the light reflex (but not the classic Argyll-Robertson pupil) has also been noted in diabetes mellitus and following trauma to the eyeball and orbit. True Argyll-Robertson pupils are small, irregular in outline, generally unequal, and lacking a response to light. In typical instances, they respond to accommodation, but the reaction may be so slight as to be difficult to see. The Argyll-Robertson pupil dilates little if at all in the dark. A poor response to painful stimuli, and only slight dilatation with mydriatics, are also characteristic. The pupillary abnormality is most commonly bilateral, although unilateral instances are found. Nonreactive dilated pupils are also occasionally encountered in luetic patients; strictly speaking they are not typically Argyll-Robertson in type and are perhaps best designated simply as "luetic pupils." The pathogenesis of the Argyll-Robertson pupil has not been well established; the responsible lesion is probably rostral to the oculomotor nucleus.

The *tonic pupil* of *Adie's syndrome* is at times confused with a luetic pupil. This disorder is unilateral in the great majority of cases. Women are more commonly affected than men. The involved pupil is generally larger than its fellow and responds poorly and slowly to light; in the dark the pupil dilates, after which it reacts to light. It responds normally to mydriatics. This pupillary disorder may be an isolated abnormality or may be associated with loss of the Achilles or patellar reflexes. Such a tonic pupil may also appear in instances of autonomic dysfunction, such as the Riley-

Day syndrome or in patients with orthostatic hypotension. The most important clinical feature of this tonic, or myotonic, pupil is its behavior on convergence. Adie states that "if the patient fixes a near object and continues to gaze at it intently, the pupil, sometimes after a delay of several seconds, contracts slowly and with increasing slowness through a range, often greatly in excess of the normal; contraction down to pinhead size is not uncommon; the large abnormal pupil then becomes smaller than its fellow." Pharmacologically, the abnormal pupil demonstrates marked hypersensitivity to the action of parasympathomimetic agents. Thus, following instillation of 2.5 percent methacholine, or 0.125 percent pilocarpine, the pupil constricts markedly, while the normal pupil fails to react. It has been suggested that the lesion responsible for this pupillary abnormality is in the ciliary ganglion, with aberrant nerve fiber regeneration.

In instances of increased intracranial pressure with herniation of the uncus of the temporal lobe through the incisura of the tentorium against the third nerve, a fixed (i.e., unresponsive to light) unilateral dilated pupil is seen, as in *Hutchinson's pupil.* This phase of dilatation, which is due to parasympathetic paralysis, is ordinarily preceded by an evanescent stage of pupillary constriction resulting from parasympathetic irritation early in the course of compression. The importance of these pupillary changes as objective evidence of herniation with increasing intracranial pressure must be emphasized. The necessity for careful observation of pupillary size under these circumstances is a strong argument against the use of mydriatics in such patients.

*Horner's syndrome* is the result of paralysis of the cervical sympathetic outflow and is characterized by contraction of the pupil, partial ptosis of the eyelid, enophthalmos, and, inconstantly, loss of sweating (i.e., anhy-

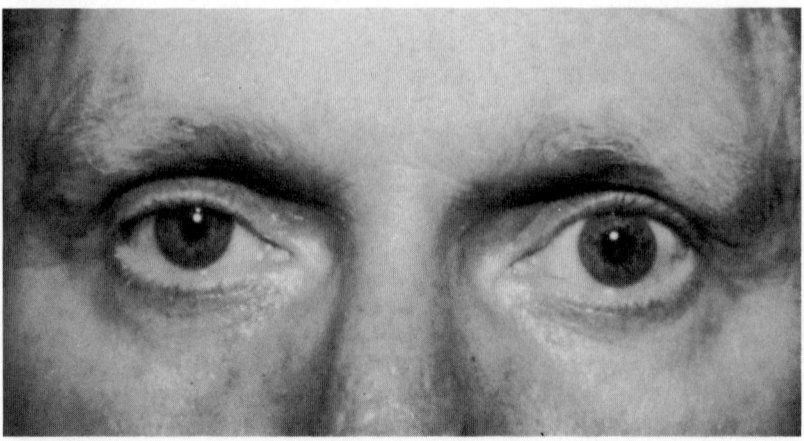

**FIGURE 2-8.** Right Horner's syndrome following cervical trauma and demonstrating ptosis and miosis.

drosis) over the affected side of the face (Fig. 2-8). It may be due to lesions affecting the cervical sympathetic trunk in the neck, such as gunshot or stab wounds, enlarged cervical nodes, tumor, or aneurysm; to both intramedullary and extramedullary lesions of the spinal cord, particularly involving the C8 and T1 segments, including tumors, meningitis, hematoma, syringomyelia, and luetic meningomyelitis; or to brainstem lesions, particularly in the medulla, such as softenings (as in the lateral medullary plate syndrome of Wallenberg), infiltrating tumors, or syringobulbia. Such brainstem lesions result in sympathetic dysfunction by virtue of involvement of the descending sympathetic pathways in the lateral tegmentum. In attempting to localize the lesion responsible for Horner's syndrome, the effect of instillation of certain pharmacologic agents into the eye may be instructive. Four percent cocaine may be used to demonstrate sympathetic paresis. A distinction between pre- and postganglionic lesions may be assisted by the use of 1 percent phenylephrine, which demonstrates pupillary hypersensitivity in postganglionic lesions. One percent hydroxyamphetamine may also be used for this purpose.

## OCULAR MOTILITY

Disturbances of movement of the eyeballs are found regularly in diseases involving the oculomotor, abducens, and trochlear nerves. These are spoken of as *ophthalmoplegias*. The nerves concerned may be affected in isolation, or in unison in the course of a host of neurologic disorders.

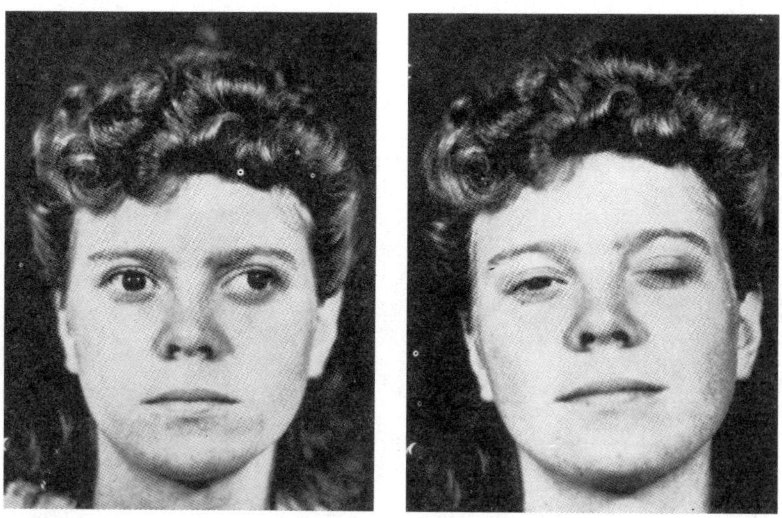

**FIGURE 2-9.** Partial ophthalmoplegia, with involvement of the left oculomotor nerve, showing ptosis of the eyelid and external strabismus in a case of cerebral aneurysm.

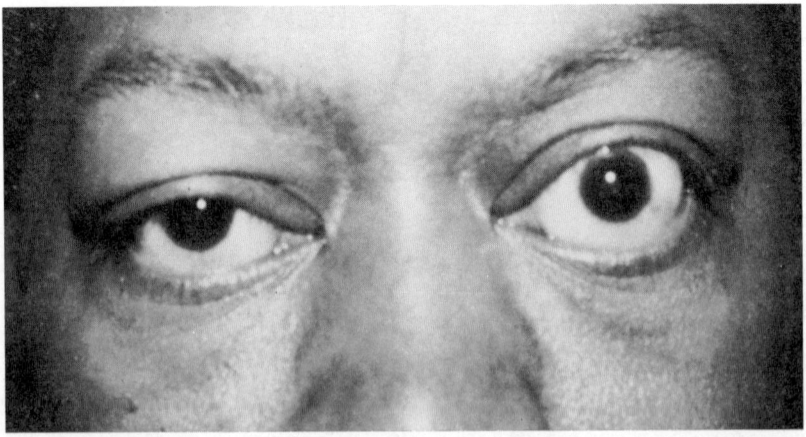

**FIGURE 2-10.** Thyroid ophthalmopathy with proptosis on the left.

They may be affected within the brainstem by involvement of their respective nuclei or of the infranuclear fiber bundles; peripherally in their course at the base of the brain; and within the orbit. Within the brainstem, they may be affected by infiltrating tumors; by demyelinating disorders, such as multiple sclerosis; by encephalitis, hemorrhage, or infarction; or by such metabolic diseases as Wernicke's encephalopathy. At the base of the brain these nerves may be involved by meningitis, especially of the more chronic granulomatous varieties; by subarachnoid hemorrhage; by compression from aneurysms of the internal carotid, posterior communicating, or posterior cerebral arteries (Fig. 2-9), or by tumors such as sphenoid ridge meningioma or intracranially extending nasopharyngeal malignancy (Schmincke tumor, Garcin's syndrome); by trauma; by metabolic disorders, such as lead poisoning or diabetes; and by mastoid disease with petrositis, affecting especially the abducens nerve *(Gradenigo syndrome).* They may also be affected by thrombosis of the cavernous sinus, through whose lateral wall they proceed, or by carotid-cavernous fistulae. In the orbit itself, the nerves may be compressed by tumor or granuloma, implicated in orbital cellulitis, or damaged in the course of orbital fractures. Finally, in any case of ocular palsy of recent onset, partial or complete, the possibility of myasthenia gravis or dysthyroid myopathy (thyroid ophthalmopathy) (Fig. 2-10) must be entertained.

## COMPLETE PARALYSIS OF ALL OCULAR NERVES

This results in ptosis of the eyelids and complete immobility of the eyeballs. When the pupils are spared, the term *external ophthalmoplegia* is applied. In *internal ophthalmoplegia,* on the other hand, the pupils are dilated and fail to react to light by virtue of paralysis of the sphincter iridis and unopposed action of the cervical sympathetics. Such an extensive paralysis of ocular movement with pupillary affection may be unilateral or bilateral, more frequently the former. It is much more likely to be the result of involvement of the nerves themselves than of their nuclei within the brainstem and is usually produced by lesions in the region of the cavernous sinus or the superior orbital fissure, where the nerves are concentrated in a small area. Meningitis, particularly of the chronic granulomatous variety, sarcoidosis, thrombosis of the cavernous sinus, tumor or aneurysm compressing the sinus, carcinomatosis of the meninges, and even the Guillain-Barré syndrome may be responsible. Complete ophthalmoplegia may also be produced by lesions within the orbit itself, or at its apex. Idiopathic granulomatous lesions at the superior orbital fissure may be responsible for a painful ophthalmoplegia referred to as the *Tolosa-Hunt syndrome.* Particular mention should be made of the occurrence of such an ophthalmoplegia in instances of lateral (parasellar) extension of a pituitary adenoma, at times developing with dramatic suddenness in the syndrome of *pituitary apoplexy.*

External ophthalmoplegia (i.e., ophthalmoplegia with sparing of the pupils) is also encountered in a variety of circumstances. It may be noted in cases of myasthenia gravis or in myotonic dystrophy and is characteristically found in progressive supranuclear palsy *(Steele-Richardson-Olszewski syndrome)* in association with dementia, muscular rigidity, dyskinesia, and pyramidal tract signs. So-called ocular myopathy, or dystrophy, sometimes also referred to as *progressive external ophthalmoplegia,* produces a more slowly evolving, ultimately total ophthalmoplegia that leaves the pupils unaffected. This curious disorder of ocular motility may be associated with other abnormalities, neurologic, ocular, muscular, and cardiac in nature; the rubric *ophthalmoplegia-plus* is sometimes applied to such instances.

Partial paralysis of the ocular nerves may occur in various combinations, and either unilaterally or bilaterally. Partial paralyses are perhaps more common with intramedullary disease and are thus often found in combination with affection of other cranial nerves, or of other intramedullary fiber systems. Although diplopia is commonly lacking in instances of complete ophthalmoplegia, it appears regularly in partial paralysis, the pattern of double vision being dependent on the particular nerves and muscles involved.

## ISOLATED PARALYSIS OF THE OCULOMOTOR (III) NERVE

*Bilateral* complete paralysis of the oculomotor nerve is rare. It may result from infarction involving the nuclei in the midbrain and is occasionally encountered in instances of multiple sclerosis or encephalitis. The eyes are held in a divergent squint, the pupils are dilated, there is bilateral ptosis, and the eyeballs cannot be moved upward, inward, or downward.

*Unilateral* paralysis of the oculomotor nerve is much more common.

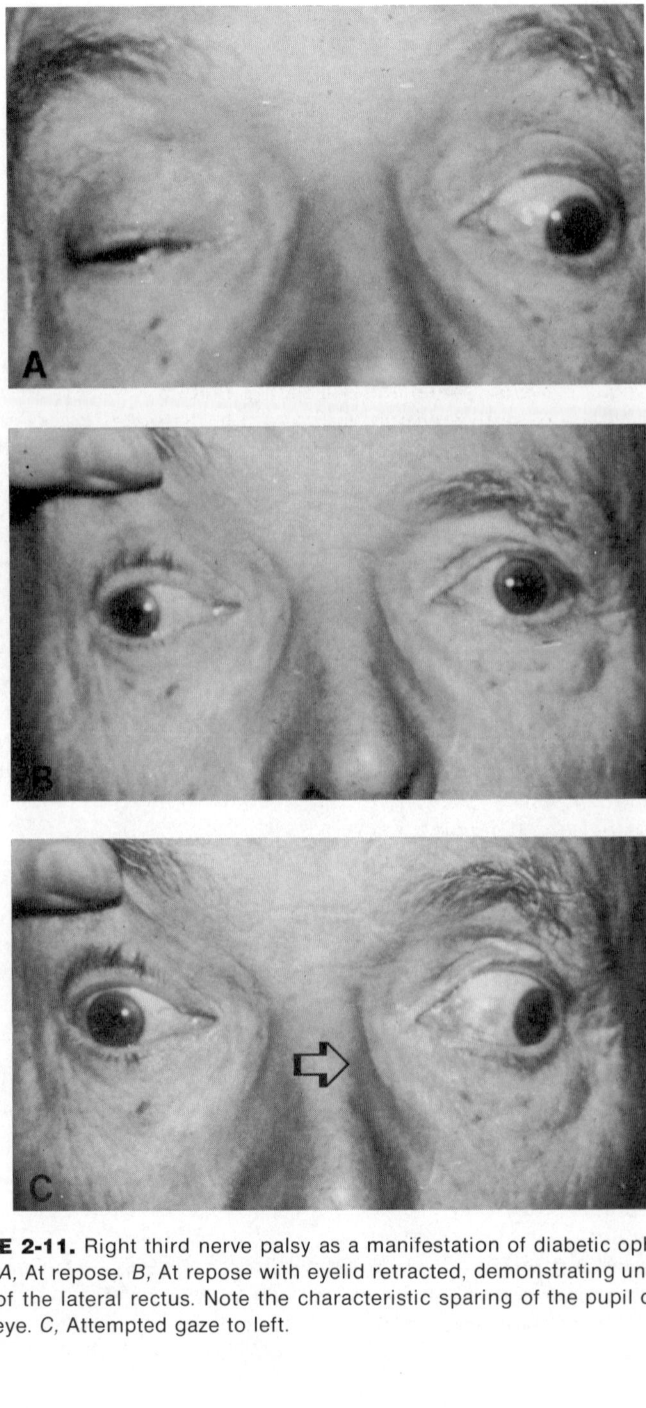


**FIGURE 2-11.** Right third nerve palsy as a manifestation of diabetic ophthalmoplegia. *A,* At repose. *B,* At repose with eyelid retracted, demonstrating unopposed action of the lateral rectus. Note the characteristic sparing of the pupil of the affected eye. *C,* Attempted gaze to left.

It is usually due to compression of the nerve in its extracerebral course as, for example, by aneurysm of the internal carotid or posterior communicating artery, by tumor of the sphenoid ridge, by lateral extension of a pituitary adenoma, by meningitis, by meningeal hemorrhage involving the nerve in the interpeduncular space, or by cranial or orbital trauma. It commonly appears as a cranial mononeuropathy in diabetes (Fig. 2-11). Unilateral oculomotor palsy may also result from intramedullary disease; thus, it is occasionally due to infarction in the mesencephalic tegmentum, along with a contralateral hemiparesis reflecting involvement of the cerebral peduncle, as in *Weber's syndrome,* or in association not only with a hemiparesis but with rubral tremor as well, as in *Benedikt's syndrome.* A unilateral *nuclear* oculomotor palsy, it should be stressed, is extremely unusual, in contrast to these affections of the intramedullary nerve fascicles. Clinically, a unilateral third nerve palsy is characterized by ptosis of the eyelid with inability to open the lid, external strabismus resulting from the unopposed action of the external rectus muscle, and inability to move the affected eyeball upward, inward, or downward. Incomplete palsies are common. The pupil is typically dilated, and the reaction of the pupil to light is generally lost. In some cases of compression of the third nerve caused by aneurysm, the pupils may escape, however, and in diabetic ophthalmoplegia the pupil is typically spared.

In the uncommon oculomotor palsy caused by a nuclear lesion, ptosis may be entirely lacking or may appear bilaterally, in contrast to that observed with involvement of the nerve itself. In such a nuclear affection a contralateral superior rectus palsy may be noted along with sparing of the ipsilateral superior rectus, a state of affairs reflecting the predominantly contralateral innervation of that muscle in the oculomotor complex.

## ISOLATED PARALYSIS OF THE TROCHLEAR (IV) NERVE

An isolated lesion involving the trochlear nerve is the least common of the isolated oculomotor palsies and is infrequently seen in a neurologic setting. It will be recalled that the trochlear nerve innervates the superior oblique muscle, moving the eyeball downward and outward; with the globe directed mesially, it is responsible for downward movement with intorsion, a movement lost in paralysis of the nerve. Tilting of the head toward the opposite shoulder is a constant accompanying sign; this posture permits binocular vision without diplopia, the latter developing as soon as the head is restored to a vertical position. When the head is tilted toward the side of the palsy, diplopia increases. Because of the head tilt, cases of trochlear paralysis are often mistaken for instances of torticollis and treated as such for some time before the correct diagnosis is established.

The most common cause of a trochlear palsy is trauma. An isolated trochlear palsy may also appear as a complication of diabetes, although less frequent than an oculomotor palsy. The nerve may also be involved by lesions within the orbit, at the orbital apex, and in the cavernous sinus. Myasthenia gravis may involve the superior oblique muscle in isolated fashion and, as with other oculomotor palsies, this diagnosis must always be entertained in the patient presenting with diplopia and ocular paresis of recent onset.

## ISOLATED PARALYSIS OF THE ABDUCENS (VI) NERVE

Since the abducens nerve innervates the external rectus muscle, paralysis of the nerve results in inability to rotate the eyeball outward. (Fig. 2-12). This is readily recognized by the internal squint that develops as a result of the unopposed action of the internal rectus. Diplopia is generally present; to avoid this, the patient tends to turn the head in the direction in which the eye muscle had been acting before onset of the deficit. The abducens nerve may be involved in either its central or peripheral portion. The nucleus may be involved in the pontine tegmentum, generally by vascular lesions (infarction); when this is the case, an ipsilateral horizontal gaze paralysis virtually always accompanies the defect because of simultaneous involvement of the pontine paramedian reticular formation. The fascicular portion of the nerve within the pons may also be involved, again particularly by infarction; under these circumstances, facial palsy, facial hypesthesia, and, at times, contralateral hemiparesis may appear, which reflect affection of contiguous structures within the pons. In its extramedullary course, the abducens nerve may be involved by a variety of lesions such as meningitis, tumor, and trauma. An isolated abducens palsy may be noted with carotid-cavernous fistula or other affections of the cavernous sinus. On occasion, individual involvement of this nerve occurs as a result of diabetes. Infection of the petrous bone in cases of mastoiditis may result in the *Gradenigo syndrome,* which comprises an ipsilateral abducens palsy associated with pain in the face and eye. Of particular importance is the appearance of abducens palsy as a nonspecific sign of increased intracranial pressure; as such it perhaps reflects the unusually long, relatively tortuous course of the nerve (it runs along the clivus, then bends sharply under the petroclinoid ligament into the cavernous sinus). As a result of its length and course, the nerve seems unusually susceptible to stretching and kinking in the face of increasing pressure from above.

Bilateral congenital abducens palsies, often associated with bilateral facial palsies, may appear on a familial basis as the *Möbius syndrome.* This is at times accompanied by a number of other congenital malformations, including skeletal deformities, hemiatrophy of the tongue, and deafness. Yet another uncommon syndrome related to abduction paralysis is *Duane's retraction syndrome,* in which retraction of the globe and narrowing of the palpebral fissure occur with attempted abduction; this perhaps reflects aberrant or anomalous innervation of the lateral rectus muscle.

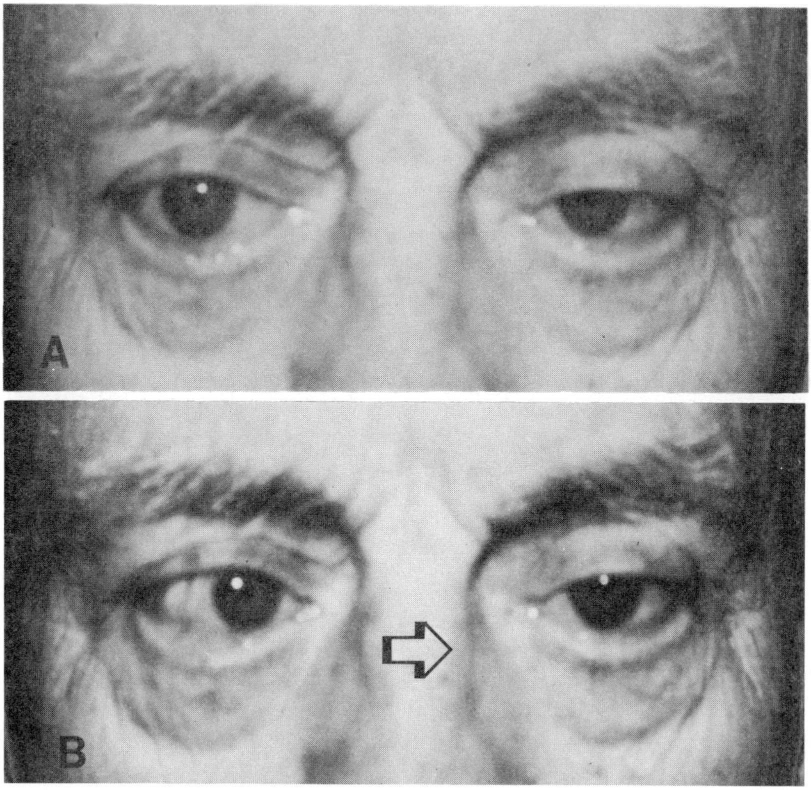

**FIGURE 2-12.** Left sixth nerve palsy due to meningeal involvement by myeloma. *A,* At repose, demonstrating unopposed action of the medial rectus muscle. *B,* Attempted gaze left, demonstrating failure of the lateral rectus.

## CONJUGATE OCULAR PARALYSIS

Paralysis of conjugate movements of the eyes occurs under diverse circumstances. Identification of such palsies is often extremely useful in localizing lesions to the brainstem or to the cerebral hemispheres. To permit full evaluation, examination should include the following: (1) volitional movements; (2) attraction movements, consisting of quick movements of the eyes toward an object in the periphery that attracts the attention; (3) following movements; and (4) segmental reflex movements (oculocephalic, caloric responses).

*Paralysis of lateral gaze* consists of inability to move the eyeballs laterally in a horizontal plane (Fig. 2-13). Defects may involve voluntary, following, or segmental reflex movements, or a combination of all three. Paralysis of lateral gaze results from a lesion in the pons, where a center is

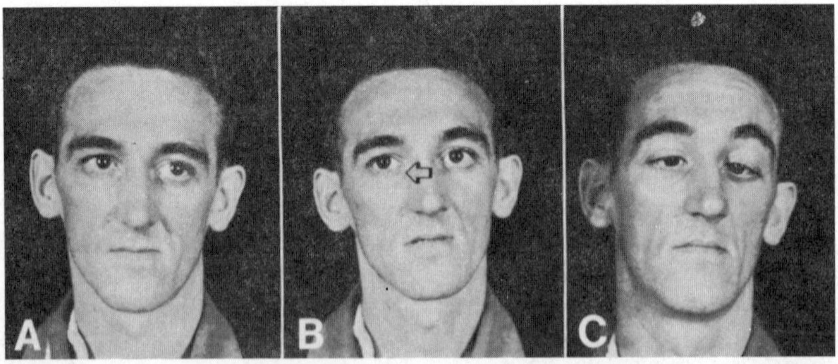

**FIGURE 2-13.** Paralysis of right lateral gaze. *A*, At repose there is gaze preference to the left. *B*, Inability to deviate eyes beyond the midline to the right. *C*, Relative preservation of convergence.

presumed to exist for such conjugate movement in the pontine paramedian reticular formation, or from involvement of the supranuclear centers for conjugate gaze in the cerebrum, located in the adversive eye field of the opposite frontal lobe and in the occipital lobe. In instances of cerebral hemispheral disease, conjugate deviation of the eyes may be encountered with either irritative or destructive lesions. In *irritative* lesions, especially those involving the frontal lobe, as in cases of a focal epileptic disorder with adversive seizures, the eyes and usually the head are deviated conjugately to the opposite side, that is, they look away from the lesion. In *destructive* lesions the gaze is directed toward the side of the lesion as a result of the unopposed action of the adversive eye field of the opposite intact hemisphere.

The distinction between supranuclear and pontine paralysis of lateral gaze is often difficult. The following points are helpful: In a lesion involving the cerebral *hemisphere,* hemiparesis almost invariably accompanies the gaze palsy. Further, in such patients, although the eyes evidence neither random nor voluntary movements, pursuit movements may be noted if the patient is alert. Additionally, in the presence of hemispheral disease, reflex eye movements can be elicited by utilizing segmental brainstem mechanisms in response to either caloric stimulation or oculocephalic (doll's head) maneuvers. In contrast, with *pontine* lesions segmental reflexes are commonly lost, as is the ability to pursue a moving object. Further, the gaze palsy with a pontine lesion is permanent, while that encountered with a cerebral hemispheral lesion is generally transitory. Finally, of course, a lesion in the pons producing a horizontal gaze palsy commonly results in other segmental neurologic signs, such as peripheral facial palsy or hemifacial sensory defect.

Bilateral hemispheral disease may result in complete loss of the ability to move the eyes in the horizontal plane; this global paralysis of horizontal gaze is sometimes called the Roth-Bielschowsky syndrome. A similar defect appears with bilateral lesions in the subthalamus and upper brainstem.

*Paralysis of upward gaze (Parinaud syndrome)* is characterized by inability to move the eyeballs vertically above the horizontal plane. It is usually although not invariably accompanied by paralysis of downward gaze. Frequently it exists without evidence of involvement of individual ocular muscles, but may be associated with changes in the pupillary reactions; only rarely is it encountered as an isolated symptom of neurologic deficit. In addition to pupillary abnormalities, the concomitant appearance of lid retraction, lid lag, failure of Bell's phenomenon, and retraction or convergence-retraction nystagmus on attempted upward movement has prompted the designation of *dorsal midbrain syndrome* as preferable to the eponym of Parinaud. Defective upward gaze appears with tumors of the pineal body compressing the midbrain tectum (collicular plate), with infiltrating tumors involving the midbrain, with infarctions, in Wernicke's encephalopathy, in association with congenital aqueductal atresia, and, albeit rarely, as a distant symptom of tumor in the cerebellopontine angle or cerebellum itself. A defect in vertical gaze may be an early manifestation of progressive supranuclear palsy (Steele-Richardson-Olszewski syndrome) (Fig. 2-14). The converse of paralysis of upward gaze, that is, forced upward gaze as typically observed in the oculogyric crises of the parkinsonian patient, presumably reflects irritation in the same anatomic region.

*Paralysis of divergence* is extremely difficult to document. It has been thought that this simply represents bilateral abducens palsies, but in true divergence paralysis, isolated lateral rectus function is said to be preserved. In addition to the divergence paralysis, such patients demonstrate homonymous diplopia; failure of increase of the angle of squint on looking to either side, but increase or decrease on looking upward and downward, which results in a tendency for the head to be held with the chin against the chest in order to promote convergence; and fusion of images being brought to within 10 to 15 inches of the patient, with development of further diplopia when the test object is moved yet closer, by virtue of a failure of convergence. The pathologic substrate for divergence paralysis is not known; it has been observed as a complication of increased intracranial pressure. Such divergence paralysis must of course be distinguished from *convergence spasm* as seen especially in hysterics.

*Paralysis of convergence* is characterized by loss of the ability of the eyeballs to converge on near objects in the face of normal function of the individual medial recti. It has been observed in encephalitis lethargica and is a characteristic abnormality in parkinsonism of both the post-encephalitic and idiopathic varieties (Fig. 2-15). It may also be encountered with infarction or demyelinative lesions involving particularly the rostal midbrain. With age, defective ocular convergence commonly appears as a normal phenomenon.

Paralysis of movement of the internal rectus muscle on lateral gaze

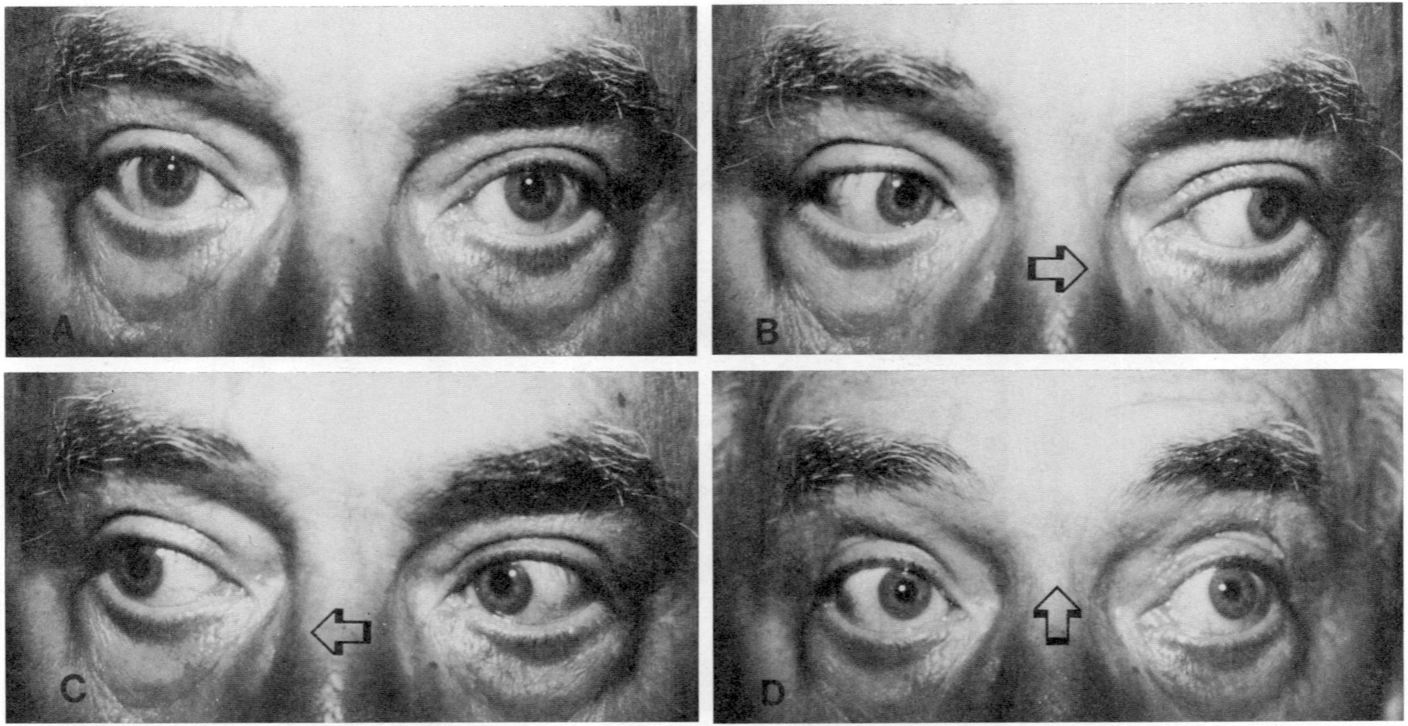


**FIGURE 2-14.** Paralysis of upward gaze in a patient with progressive supranuclear palsy. Gaze to either side is preserved. *A*, At repose. *B*, Gaze left. *C*, Gaze right. *D*, Attempted upward gaze.

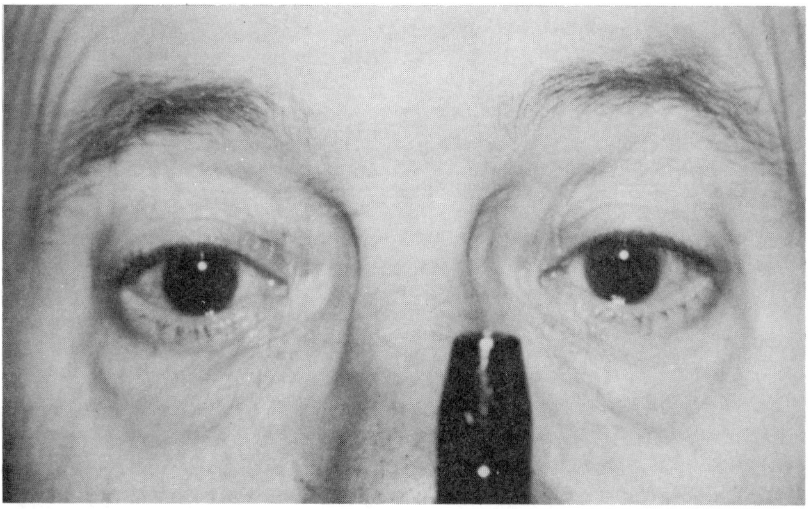

**FIGURE 2-15.** Failure of ocular convergence in a patient with paralysis agitans.

with retention of convergence is designated as *internuclear ophthalmoplegia* (INO) and is due to a lesion involving the medial longitudinal fasciculus. Characteristically accompanying the paralysis of adduction (Fig. 2-16) is monocular nystagmus of the abducting eye (ataxic nystagmus). INO is observed most commonly in instances of multiple sclerosis, but may be seen in instances of infarction and, rarely, in cases of brainstem tumor. The disorder may be unilateral or bilateral. At times, a lesion will involve both the medial longitudinal fasciculus and the pontine paramedian reticular formation on the same side. As a result, the patient exhibits not only an internuclear ophthalmoplegia on gaze to the opposite side, but an ipsilateral horizontal gaze palsy as well; this has been called the $1\frac{1}{2}$ *syndrome.*

## Trigeminal (V)

The trigeminal nerve is composed of both motor and sensory portions. In disease processes involving this cranial nerve, motor and sensory dysfunction may appear in isolated fashion or in combination. In terms of manifestations of abnormality referable to the *motor* portion of the nerve, atrophy of the affected masseter, pterygoid, and temporal muscles can be detected generally by direct palpation of the muscles; weakness can be demonstrated as previously described. The deviation of the jaw is to the paralyzed side when the mouth is open, and because of this deflection, the tongue appears to deviate as well. This is a spurious impression, however, since a line drawn through the incisors will be found to cut through the tip of the tongue. Uncommonly, hypertrophy of the muscles

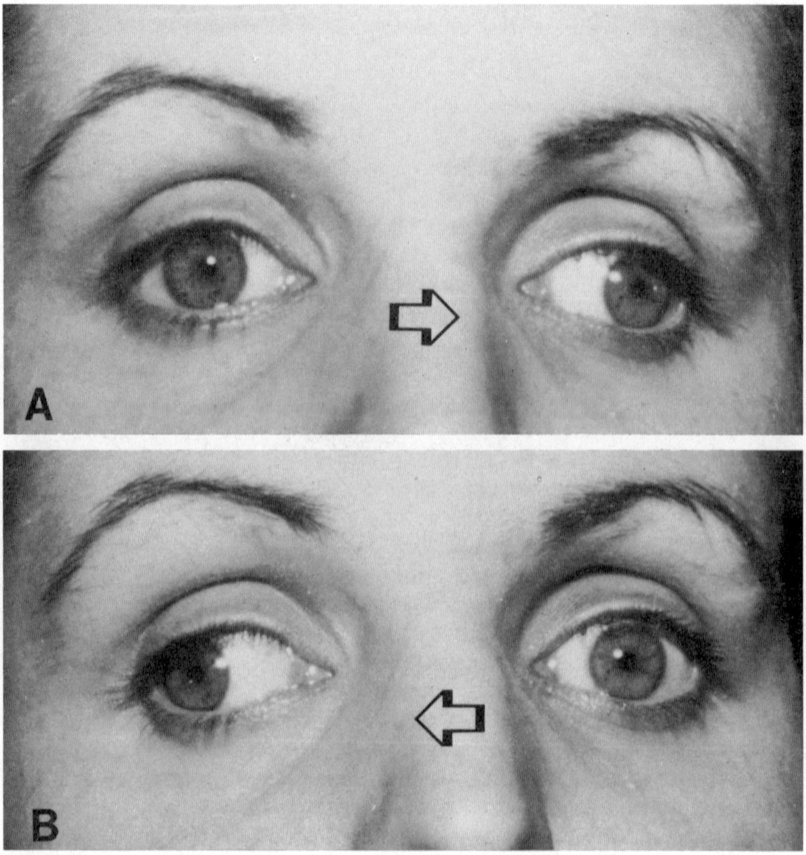


**FIGURE 2-16.** Internuclear ophthalmoplegia, demonstrating failure of adduction on gaze left *(A)* and gaze right *(B)*.

innervated solely by the trigeminal nerve is found, without accompanying weakness, as in the syndrome of benign hypertrophy of the masseters, or *hypertrophic branchial myopathy.* The cause of this disorder, which does not appear related to more generalized myopathies, is not known.

Weakness and atrophy of the muscles supplied by the trigeminal nerve not uncommonly result from a peripheral lesion such as skull fracture or tumor. The nerve may be compressed at its exit from the pons by a tumor in the cerebellopontine angle or may be involved within the brainstem by infiltrating tumor or softening involving either the motor nucleus of the nerve or its intramedullary fascicular portion.

The *sensory* division of the trigeminal nerve supplies the face and the head to the vertex, the cornea, and the mucuous membranes of the nose, mouth, hard and soft palate, and tongue to the midline. Complete interruption of sensory function is rare, but may be observed with tumors involving the gasserian ganglion, as in meningioma of Meckel's cave, or with inflammatory disease of the ganglion, such as herpes zoster. In such instances it is associated with pain in the face along the branches of the trigeminal nerve. Incomplete sensory syndromes involving the face are found in infiltrating tumors of the brainstem, or with other conditions that affect the central sensory connections of the trigeminal nerve, such as infarction or multiple sclerosis. In general, the sensory loss under these circumstances is in the distribution of one or another of the classic peripheral divisions of the nerve (Fig. 2-17). There is reversal of representation in the descending (spinal) root of the trigeminal: the ophthalmic division (VI) is represented most inferiorly, the mandibular (V3) and maxillary (V2) divisions more superiorly. Lesions higher in the tract in the brainstem may thus give rise to a sensory deficit over the lower face, while a lesion low in the medulla, or even in the upper cervical cord, may be associated with sensory loss over the forehead. A special variety of sensory alteration may be encountered with lesions of the descending root: at times, the sensory loss appears to follow a so-called onion-peel arrangement that does not correspond to the accustomed anatomic zones in the periphery (Fig. 2-18).

Direct involvement of the peripheral branches of the trigeminal nerve may arise in many situations, including tumor, infection such as herpes zoster, and trauma. Involvement of the ophthalmic division with disease

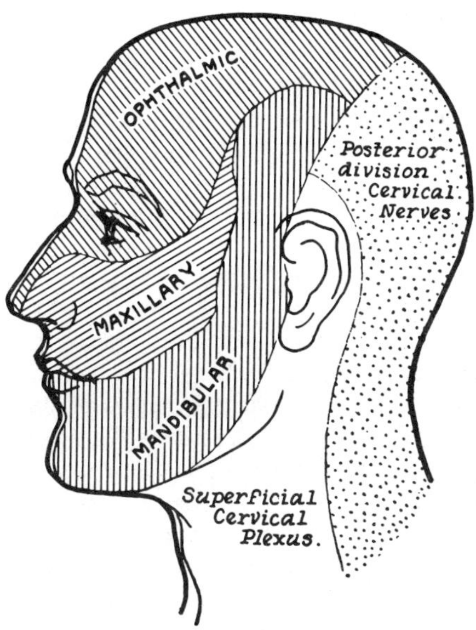


**FIGURE 2-17.** Trigeminal nerve, showing the areas of supply of the three principal divisions.

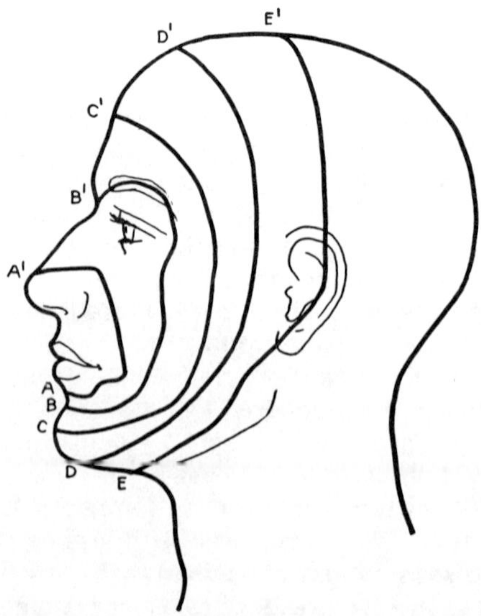


**FIGURE 2-18.** Trigeminal nerve, showing the type of onion-peel sensory loss (pain and temperature) found in lesions within the brainstem affecting the descending root of the trigeminal nerve.

of the cavernous sinus may cause sensory deficit with pain in an appropriate distribution, which appears in association with ophthalmoplegia and, at times, proptosis and chemosis.

An early manifestation of sensory loss in the distribution of the trigeminal nerve is impairment of the corneal reflex. In fact, this may be the only evidence of involvement of the sensory branch. It occurs early in many cases of cerebellopontine angle tumor and is usually the first sign of neural dysfunction beyond the auditory nerve itself under such circumstances. It may also be found in cases of hemiplegia, in infiltrating tumors of the pons, in encephalitis, in demyelinating diseases, in tumors or viral infections involving the gasserian ganglion, in herpes zoster ophthalmicus, following section of the trigeminal nerve for trigeminal neuralgia, and, in brief, in any disorder affecting the sensory nucleus of the trigeminal nerve in the brainstem, the nerve fascicles themselves (either intra- or extra-axially), the gasserian ganglion, or even with local disease of the globe.

Although the trigeminal nerve plays an important role in autonomic function, abnormalities in this sphere are only rarely encountered with trigeminal nerve dysfunction. A Horner's syndrome in association with facial pain may, however, be encountered as the so-called *paratrigeminal syndrome,* which is usually due to extramedullary tumor or aneurysm.

## Facial (VII)

Involvement of the facial nerve occurs frequently in diseases of the nervous system. Careful distinction must be made between central and peripheral nerve involvement.

*Central* facial weakness is characterized by weakness of movement of the lower portion of the face on the side opposite the lesion; movements of the frontalis are preserved. This sparing is due to the fact that the frontalis receives innervation from both motor areas, whereas the lower facial muscles are innervated only from the opposite motor cortex (Fig. 2-19). A central, or supranuclear, facial paresis is recognized by a slight drooping of the corner of the mouth and upper lip on the affected side during repose, along with widening of the palpebral fissure, and flattening of the nasolabial fold with weakness in voluntary retraction of the corner of the mouth on the affected side. Slight differences may be difficult to recognize, and mild facial assymetry on a congenital basis is a common source of confusion. In the usual case of central facial weakness the forehead can be wrinkled normally and closure of the eyelid is normal. In acute cases, however, some frontalis weakness may be seen; in such instances, the weakness in the lower portion of the face is always more pronounced, while that of the upper portion tends to disappear within a few days. While voluntary facial expression is thus weak in central facial palsies caused by a hemispheral lesion, emotional expression often remains intact. In lesions of the thalamus, on the other hand, emotional expression may be lost while voluntary movements are preserved. This

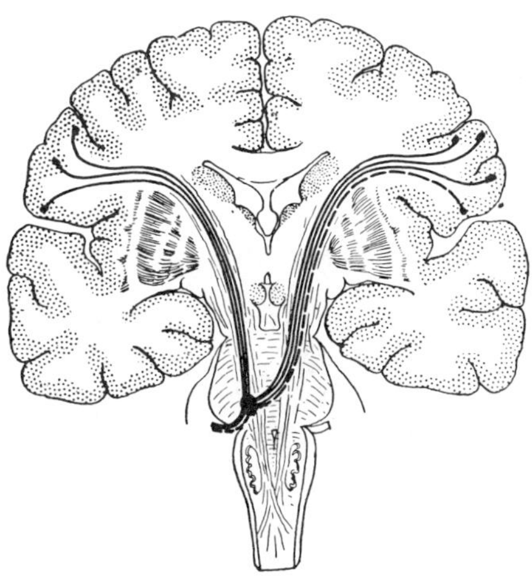

**FIGURE 2-19.** Bilateral innervation of the upper portion of the facial nerve (solid lines) and unilateral innervation of the lower portion (broken lines), which accounts for sparing of the frontalis muscle in central facial weakness.

dissociation of voluntary and emotional expression may be useful in differentiating a deep-seated from a cortical lesion.

A central facial palsy results from lesions involving the motor innervation to the face anywhere between the area representing the face in the opposite motor cortex and the nucleus of the facial nerve in the pons. It may be isolated or it may be associated with weakness of the hand, arm, or other parts of the body. Central facial weakness alone, or with other focal weakness (faciobrachial monoplegia), may be the result of a relatively small focal lesion of the opposite motor cortex, but may equally be a residual of an old, more extensive hemiparesis or hemiplegia. Indeed, in most instances central facial weakness is associated with hemiparesis and reflects simultaneous interruption of corticospinal and corticobulbar pathways by a wide variety of pathologic processes.

*Peripheral* facial paralysis differs from central facial weakness by virtue of involvement of all portions of the facial musculature. It results from a lesion of the facial nerve anywhere in its peripheral course from the facial nucleus in the pons to its distribution in the face. The lesion producing the paralysis is ipsilateral to the paralysis. All portions of the face on the affected side are paralyzed. Wrinkling of the forehead, closure of the eyelid, and movements of the muscles of facial expression are impossible. The nerve trunks on the face may be tender. Peripheral facial

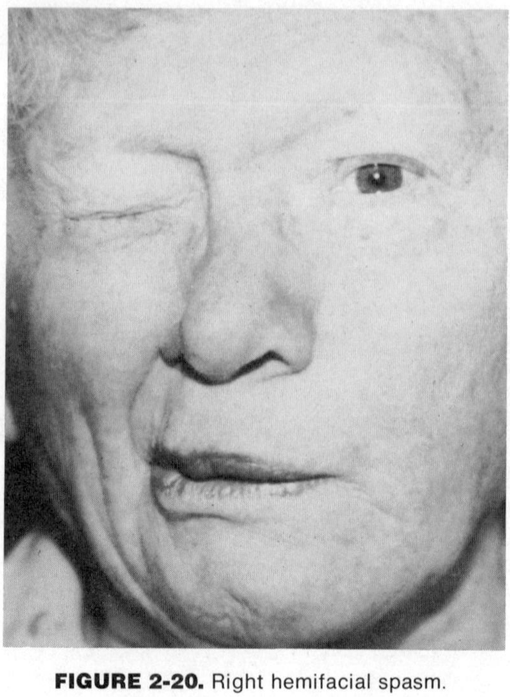

**FIGURE 2-20.** Right hemifacial spasm.

paralysis may result from involvement of the facial nucleus itself or of the intramedullary portion of the nerve in the pons, as in poliomyelitis, motor system disease, encephalitis, softening, or infiltrating glioma. The nerve may also be affected in its extracerebral intracranial course by cerebellopontine angle tumors, granulomatous meningitis, or subarachnoid hemorrhage, and seems especially liable to be involved in sarcoidosis. The nerve may also be involved at any point in its course through the petrous bone, or after its emergence from the skull, as the result, for example, of basal skull fracture, Paget's disease, mastoiditis, diabetes, or herpes zoster (as in the Ramsay-Hunt syndrome of geniculate herpes). Parotid gland tumors or surgery upon the parotid may also result in facial paralysis. The paralysis resulting from involvement of the facial nucleus itself is characterized by signs of anterior horn cell involvement, in particular fasciculations, and atrophy of the facial musculature may appear. When the nerve is diseased within the mastoid canal, as in instances of Bell's palsy, a loss of taste over the anterior two thirds of the tongue is typically found. Alterations in hearing may also be noted, which reflects involvement of the nerve to the stapedius.

*Hemifacial spasm,* that is, uncontrollable and irregular muscular contractions of variable amplitude that are limited to one side of the face (Fig. 2-20) or to a portion thereof, may develop following a Bell's palsy, but may also reflect nuclear disease; in many patients the cause is never identified.

## Acoustic (VIII)

The acoustic nerve is composed of *cochlear* and *vestibular* divisions; the former is concerned with hearing, the latter with equilibrium. Disease of the cochlea is characterized by a nerve or sensorineural type of hearing loss, the main features of which are loss or impairment of hearing, equal air and bone conduction thresholds on the audiogram, and decreased speech intelligibility scores. There is usually, but not invariably, an associated history of *tinnitus,* at times present for some time before the hearing loss itself ensues. Tinnitus is usually the result of disease of the end organ and thus associated with middle or inner ear disease or with disease of the peripheral portions of the auditory nerve. Only rarely does it develop as a consequence of involvement of the central projections of the auditory nerve in the brainstem, or higher. The constancy and quality of the tinnitus itself are unfortunately of no help in distinguishing clinically a peripheral from a central lesion.

Nerve deafness virtually always results from disease of the peripheral portion of the auditory nerve and thus may reflect acoustic neurinoma, meningioma *en plaque,* other tumors in the vicinity of the cerebellopontine angle, granulomatous meningitis, Paget's disease of the skull, or basal skull fracture, among other causes. Theoretically, it may occur as a result of central lesions involving the auditory pathways in the brainstem and their termination in the temporal lobes. In actuality, however, this occurs extremely rarely, since the auditory pathways are both crossed and uncrossed; a very extensive lesion would therefore be required to cause loss of hearing—so extensive, in fact, as to render the patient incapacitated as far as appropriate testing is concerned. Loss of hearing can most accurately be assessed by routine and special audiometric testing. Simply put, notes of standard frequency and varying intensities are sent through the ear, and nerve deafness is indicated most often by a loss of hearing, particularly in the higher frequencies. A special form of hearing disturbance is found in *Ménière's disease,* which comprises a fluctuating sensorineural loss, a "roaring" type tinnitus in the affected ear, and loudness recruitment, in addition to vertigo; ultimately, severe loss of hearing supervenes.

The vestibular portion of the auditory nerve is frequently affected in diseases of the nervous system. The outstanding subjective complaint is one of vertigo, a symptom, as already noted, that requires careful analysis.

## NYSTAGMUS

### Definition

Nystagmus is the pre-eminent objective manifestation of such disorders. Both vertigo and nystagmus are, under these circumstances, commonly associated with a sense of imbalance and dysequilibrium, and at times frank ataxia, which are generally precipitated, or intensified, by sudden changes in position of the head and neck. Nystagmus itself is thus a feature of disorders involving the vestibular portion of the auditory nerve and its central connections and may be found under a host of circumstances. By virtue of its importance in neurologic diagnosis, a detailed consideration of its features is desirable at this point.

Nystagmus may be defined most simply as an involuntary oscillation of the eyeball(s). It is usually bilateral, the two eyes moving synchronously, but unilateral disconjugate nystagmus may occur. Nystagmus may be rhythmic or pendular. In pendular nystagmus, there are more or less regular to and fro movements of equal range and velocity. In rhythmic nystagmus, on the other hand, one observes alternate slow and fast ocular movements; the rapid (saccadic) movement is in the direction of gaze and is followed by a slower return movement. Nystagmus is traditionally named after the direction of the fast component. Typically, the intensity of the nystagmus increases with gaze toward the fast phase (Alexander's law).

Nystagmus may be horizontal, vertical, oblique, rotary, or mixed in form and may be directed toward either side, upward, or downward. The rate of movements varies from 10 to 1000 oscillations/min. It may be transient or sustained, spontaneous or induced, congenital or acquired, and may be present at rest, on fixation, or on deviation of the eyeballs.

## Classification

Many classifications have been utilized in attempting to clarify the problem of nystagmus. A common grouping, for example, is into ocular, vestibular, and central types. It may also be graded on the basis of severity, with first degree (nystagmus present only on gaze to one side), second degree (present on gaze to one side and directly ahead), and third degree (present on gaze to both sides, as well as straight ahead). The approach utilized here follows Cogan in most particulars (Table 2-2); it has the advantage of being based directly on the characteristics of the movements as they are seen by the examiner.

**PENDULAR NYSTAGMUS.** The movements in pendular nystagmus are oscillating, almost always horizontal, and approximately equal in both directions. Only one eye may be involved and under these circumstances the movements may be vertical. Head nodding may accompany the eye movement. When the patient looks to either side, jerk (rhythmic) nystagmus appears with the fast component in the direction of gaze. Impairment of central vision is a hallmark of the pendular variety of nystagmus; the worse the vision, the coarser are the movements. Pendular nystagmus is characteristically encountered in individuals with vision defective from birth or infancy, or in those with defective fixation. If vision is lost after the age of 6 years, no such movements occur. The term "searching" is sometimes applied to this form of nystagmus and implies that the eyes are moving to compensate for the central scotoma that is generally present; this does not seem to be the case, however, and the movements more likely result from failure of normal tonic innervation of the ocular muscles

**TABLE 2-2.** Principle forms of nystagmus

- PENDULAR (OSCILLATING) NYSTAGMUS
    - Congenital with visual defect
    - Occupational
    - Spasmus nutans
    - Voluntary
- JERK (RHYTHMIC) NYSTAGMUS
    - Optokinetic
    - Labyrinthine (vestibular)
    - Neuromuscular
        - Paretic
        - Fatigue
        - Eccentric fixation
    - Congenital
    - Latent
    - Positional
    - See-Saw
    - Downbeat

from the macula. Many conditions are associated with pendular nystagmus, including infantile macular chorioretinitis, albinism with faulty development of the macula, total color blindness, congenital cataract, ophthalmia neonatorum, interstitial keratitis, congenital corneal leukoma, and high-grade infantile myopia.

Several subvarieties of pendular nystagmus may be isolated:

**Occupational Nystagmus.** This is an oscillating, fine, rapid, and often vertical nystagmus, which is increased on upward gaze. Fixation is defective. It is seen typically in miners and in others who work in poor light for long periods, such as compositors, draftsmen, or jewelers.

**Spasmus Nutans.** Usually associated with head nodding, and either monocular or binocular, this form of pendular nystagmus is rapid and often asymmetrical, varying with different directions of gaze. It generally appears within the first 2 years of life and ordinarily disappears spontaneously. Although sometimes likened to occupational nystagmus, its cause is unknown.

**Voluntary Nystagmus.** Some individuals are able to induce very rapid horizontal oscillating movements of the eyes voluntarily. Fixation, convergence, or widening of the palpebral fissures may increase the movements. Similar movements, associated with rigid fixation of the head, may be seen in tense, neurotic individuals.

**JERK NYSTAGMUS (RHYTHMIC NYSTAGMUS).** In this form of nystagmus the movements are unequal, and both fast and slow components can be recognized. As already indicated, the nystagmus is named after the fast component, even though this is not necessarily primary pathogenically. Typically the intensity of nystagmus increases when gaze is aimed in the direction of the fast phase.

**Optokinetic Nystagmus.** Generally rather fine and rapid, this form of nystagmus is elicited by rotating a drum or tape with regularly spaced vertical stripes before the eyes; it also occurs when a patient in a rapidly moving vehicle directs his eyes on fixed objects (railroad or elevator nystagmus). The slow, or following, phase is in the direction of rotation of the drum. Defective horizontal opticokinetic responses, or absence of them, are most commonly encountered with lesions in the posterior half of the cerebral hemispheres when the drum is rotated to the side of the lesion. The abnormality may be seen with or without an associated hemianopic defect. More anteriorly placed lesions are uncommonly associated with this alteration. Bilateral reduction in opticokinetic responses is sometimes found, but cannot be correlated accurately with lesions in a particular location. It should be pointed out that since the slow, following phase of opticokinetic nystagmus is initiated by visual cues, this form of nystagmus may be used as a crude guide to visual function, even in newborns. It also has widespread application in this respect to malingerers, hysterics, aphasics, and retarded and obtunded individuals. Opticokinetic nystagmus is also of assistance in documenting subtle ocular palsies, in which impairment of movement is most obvious on inspection of the fast, or saccadic, phase.

**Labyrinthine (Vestibular) Nystagmus.** Characteristically, nystagmus of this type follows stimulation of the semicircular canal and results from movement of the endolymph with stimulation of the vestibular nerves. It is characterized by the presence of both slow and fast components and may be looked upon as a reflex response to movements of the head or body, or to direct stimulation of the labyrinth. It may be horizontal, rotary, or both. Rotation in a Bárány chair, thermal (caloric) stimulation, and galvanic excitation may all be utilized to produce this form of nystagmus. Labyrinthine nystagmus may also occur spontaneously in disease of the labyrinthine apparatus itself, or of the vestibular nuclei; spontaneous rotary nystagmus is especially common with lesions affecting the latter structures. When the nystagmus is due to a lesion of the labyrinth (as in labyrinthitis or Ménière's disease), or of the eighth nerve, vertigo, tinnitus, and alteration of hearing are frequent, whereas with central lesions these are uncommon. Loss of response to caloric stimuli is found with nuclear lesions, a feature of major importance in locating the site of involvement. Many pathologic processes involve the vestibular nuclei and are thus capable of producing labyrinthine nystagmus; among the more common are softening caused by occlusive vascular disease, multiple sclerosis, Wernicke's encephalopathy, and mass lesions in the cerebellum or cerebellopontine angle. Lesions that involve the medial longitudinal fasciculus (MLF) (multiple sclerosis, infarction) produce predominantly monocular ataxic nystagmus as part of the syndrome of internuclear ophthalmoplegia, which consists of weakness of the medial rectus on conjugate lateral gaze with nystagmus of labyrinthine type in the abducting eye. As previously noted, this may be either unilateral or bilateral. The nystagmus that may appear in association with lesions of the upper cervical cord may reflect involvement of the lowermost projection of the MLF.

A variety of chemical substances may produce spontaneous labyrinthine nystagmus or alter induced labyrinthine responses; among these are barbiturates, phenytoin, quinine, and streptomycin.

In severe instances of labyrinthine nystagmus, the patient may experience a sensation of illusory movement of the environment; this is called *oscillopsia.* Curiously, however, in most instances of nystagmus the patient appears unaware of the actual movement of the eyeballs.

**Nystagmus Caused by Neuromuscular Insufficiency.** Unsustained nystagmoid jerks are seen in a large number of normal individuals on extreme deviation of the eyes. This is referred to as *end-point* nystagmus and is of no clinical significance. Exaggeration of this type of nystagmus is seen in the following:

1. Paretic nystagmus, which develops on attempted use of a paretic ocular muscle. It may occur with gaze palsies as well.

2. Fatigue nystagmus, which follows excessive use or increased fatigability of certain ocular muscles.

3. Nystagmus of eccentric fixation. This occurs on deviation of the eyes beyond the limits of the binocular field. It is jerky and occurs in 50 to 60 percent of normal individuals.

**Congenital Nystagmus.** This dates from birth and is sometimes inherited. It must be differentiated from pendular nystagmus, which does not develop until fixation is attempted. Defective opticokinetic responses may be found.

**Latent Nystagmus.** This appears on covering one eye in subjects with poor visual acuity or without binocular vision, especially patients with amblyopia that results from strabismus. It occurs in the covered eye and is in the direction of the open eye. The cause is unknown.

**Positional Nystagmus.** Often associated with a complaint of vertigo, this variety of nystagmus has special significance. It is induced as follows: the patient sits on a table with the head turned to one side and the gaze fixed on the examiner's head. The examiner grasps the patient's head and pushes him back briskly into the supine position with the head below the level of the table and rotated 30 to 45 degrees to one side. If nystagmus occurs the head is held in this position for 30 seconds, after which the patient is brought upright, and the test is repeated with the head turned to the opposite side. In the fatigable type the nystagmus appears after a latency of 2 to 10 seconds and subsides in 5 to 30 seconds. In the nonfatigable form the nystagmus appears without latency, as soon as the head is placed in the critical position, and persists as long as this position is maintained. The fatigable type of positional nystagmus is most common with lesions of the end organ and is often found after head injuries; the nonfatigable form tends to occur with centrally placed lesions.

**See-saw Nystagmus.** A rare form of nystagmus, this is characterized by rotary (tortional) movements of the eyes along with dissociated and simultaneous vertical movements; as one eye moves up, the other eye moves down, and vice versa. It most commonly occurs in cases of supersellar tumors that involve the third ventricle, but may result from softening in the upper brainstem.

**Downbeat Nystagmus.** This is a rhythmic nystagmus with a fast component directed downward, which is elicited by looking downward and often exaggerated when looking to the side and down. It generally indicates a lesion in the vicinity of the foramen magnum, as is encountered with the Arnold-Chiari syndrome. The reverse, *upbeat nystagmus,* is a coarse nystagmus that increases when gaze is directed upward and appears in at least some instances to be related to a lesion in the cerebellar vermis.

## Other Abnormal Eye Movements

Several varieties of abnormal eye movements are sometimes confused with nystagmus and require careful differentiation. These may be enumerated as follows:

1. *Opsoclonus* consists of irregular, nonrhythmic, lightning-like jerking movements of the eyes encountered in comatose patients with lesions of the brainstem. Movements of this sort also occur in association with cerebellar ataxia in patients with neuroblastoma and may be seen in instances of the postinfectious ataxic syndrome in children.

2. *Ocular myoclonus* is a syndrome of regular, rhythmic, quick, and usually conjugate to-and-fro movements of the eyes, with a frequency of 120 to 140 beats/min, which is associated with synchronous movements of the palate and, on occasion, other bulbar muscles. Such movements may appear in bursts, often triggered by eyelid closure or by horizontal gaze movements. It generally follows a lesion, usually softening, which interrupts the dentato-rubro-olivary circuit, particularly in a paramedian distribution in the pons; a pretectal localization has also been suggested.

3. *Ocular dysmetria,* or ocular past-pointing, is overshooting of the line of vision when the eyes are directed quickly to a target; it is found in patients with cerebellar disease and is analogous to hypermetria (past-pointing) of the limbs.

4. *Oculogyric crises* are found most commonly in instances of post-encephalitic parkinsonism, but may be found in the idiopathic form as well. These consist of attacks of involuntary, forced, upward deviation of the eyes, which at times are temporarily controllable with maximal voluntary effort.

5. *Ocular cogwheeling* is a curious, jerky, irregular movement of the eyeballs sometimes observed in parkinsonian patients on horizontal gaze. It is thought to be analogous to the cogwheeling observed on passive movements of the limbs.

6. *Ocular bobbing* is a term referring to the appearance of abrupt, spontaneous, conjugate vertical eye movements, which are generally associated with a loss of lateral movements of the eyes and most commonly encountered in comatose individuals. The predominant rapid movement is downward, with a slow drift to the midposition. This phenomenon is generally attributed to vascular lesions within the pontine tegmentum, with resultant dissociation of vertical from lateral movements.

7. *Nystagmus retractorius* consists of jerk-like retraction movements of the globes, commonly rhythmic, usually bilateral, and occurring either spontaneously or in response to eye movements. Ocular palsies, especially

of upward gaze, may be found. The responsible lesion appears to be in the periaqueductal region of the midbrain.

## Glossopharyngeal (IX)

A lesion involving the glossopharyngeal nerve is characterized by loss of taste over the posterior third of the tongue and impaired sensation over the palate and pharynx. This has been observed in granulomatous meningitis; in infiltrating tumors of the brainstem or of the base of the skull that implicate the jugular foramen; and with basal skull fractures. Pain in the throat is characteristically encountered in *glossopharyngeal neuralgia,* a rare disease characterized by severe paroxysms of pain initiated by swallowing. As regards motor function, the glossopharyngeal nerve innervates the stylopharyngeus muscle, which elevates and widens the pharynx on swallowing; impairment is ordinarily not recognizable clinically.

## Vagus (X)

The vagus is an extremely long nerve that may be affected in the medulla, at the base of the skull, within the jugular foramen, in the neck or thorax, or even in the abdomen. Generally speaking, from the standpoint of motor function the vagus supplies the musculature of the larynx, pharynx, and palate (external laryngeal, recurrent laryngeal, pharyngeal nerves) and also supplies visceral motor fibers to the heart, lungs, and alimentary tract. Additionally, it carries sensory information from the pharynx, larynx, epiglottis, trachea, esophagus, heart, lungs, stomach, and small intestine. Symptoms of deficit vary considerably, depending upon the point at which the nerve is involved. From a practical viewpoint, disturbances of swallowing and of phonation are the most important and perhaps most easily recognized.

Within the lower brainstem itself, the nerve may be involved by processes such as infiltrating gliomas, infarction (particularly with occlusive disease involving the posterior inferior cerebellar artery), syringobulbia, poliomyelitis, multiple sclerosis, or motor system disease. At the base of the brain it may be affected by granulomatous meningitis; by tumors, either within the cranial vault or involving the skull itself, particularly at the jugular foramen; and by fractures at the base. In its cervical portion, the nerve may be injured by stab or gunshot wounds or may be damaged during operations upon the thyroid; tumors and aneurysms of the carotid or subclavian arteries may also compress the nerve. Finally, a variety of mediastinal lesions including enlarged lymph nodes, neoplasm, or aneurysms of the aorta itself may involve the nerve.

*Aphonia,* or hoarseness, may result from involvement of the nucleus ambiguus itself, or of the infranuclear fibers of the vagus as they course through the medulla or the posterior fossa, or from isolated affection of the recurrent laryngeal nerve. It is associated with abductor paralysis of the vocal cord, which may be unilateral or bilateral. In the former, hoarseness is present; in the latter, the voice is lost entirely, and dyspnea and stridorous respirations may ensue.

*Dysphagia* (weakness or paralysis of swallowing) is noted under a variety of circumstances. It may be found in patients with hemiplegia in association with palatal weakness, or it may result from involvement of the muscles of deglutition caused by a nuclear lesion that involves the nucleus ambiguus, but it may also appear with bilateral supranuclear lesions, as in pseudobulbar palsy. In such instances the palate moves poorly, if at all, and there is loss of power of the middle and inferior constrictors of the pharynx. Regurgitation of liquids through the nose occurs as a result of inability to close the pharynx when swallowing. In some instances of dysphagia the palate is capable of moving well, but the inferior pharyngeal constrictions fail to function; loss of function of the latter is evidenced by weakness or loss of movement of the Adam's apple on attempted swallowing.

Along with these difficulties in speaking and swallowing, lesions of the vagus may also be expressed by loss of the palatal and pharyngeal reflexes and by impairment of sensation in the external auditory meatus and the pinna.

## Spinal Accessory (XI)

The spinal accessory nerve is uncommonly involved in isolation. It may be injured by gunshot or stab wounds in the neck, by surgical procedures in the neck, by fracture dislocation of the cervical vertebrae, by a variety of tumors in the vicinity of the foramen magnum or at the base of the brain, by vertebral artery aneurysm, and by a host of intramedullary disorders, such as syringobulbia, motor system disease, or poliomyelitis. Paralysis of the sternocleidomastoid muscle is characterized by flatness of the neck on the affected side, with failure of the muscle to stand out on rotation of the neck and weakness during this maneuver. When only one sternomastoid is affected, the resting posture of the head remains unchanged; when both sternocleidomastoid muscles are paralyzed, however, there is decided weakness of flexion of the head on the neck. With involvement of the trapezius, flattening of the normal contour of the muscle may be seen, along with a dropped shoulder. Weakness is observed when the patient attempts to shrug the shoulder, and there is difficulty in raising the arm above the horizontal plane. The scapula tends to be rotated slightly downward and outward; in severe instances mild winging of the scapula may be seen.

## Hypoglossal (XII)

The hypoglossal nerve, like the facial, may show evidence of central or peripheral involvement. Often overlooked, central (i.e., supranuclear) weakness of the hypoglossal nerve is characterized by deviation of the tongue to the affected (i.e., hemiparetic) side. Atrophy and fasciculations are lacking. In instances of peripheral (nuclear or infranuclear) palsy, the tongue deviates to the side of the lesion, and atrophy and fasciculations are characteristically encountered (Fig. 2-21). In early cases, the atrophy can be detected as an indentation or scalloping along the edges of the tongue. A search for fasciculations is expedited by investigating the tongue at rest on the floor of the mouth, since protrusion of the tongue may at times result in obscuration of these involuntary movements, while at the same time be responsible for the appearance of potentially confusing tremulousness in many individuals. As the responsible lesion becomes more advanced, atrophy is increasingly apparent as the tongue shrinks perceptibly on the affected side. With the tongue in the floor of the mouth, curvature is seen toward the healthy side. Fasciculations are active and easily seen when the process is well developed; the tongue is in a state of lively motion resembling a "bag of worms." In severe cases, particularly with bilateral palsy, the tongue cannot be protruded. A number of lesions in the lower brainstem may result in such peripheral affection, including syringobulbia, motor system disease, infiltrating glioma, and infarction. Inability to protrude the tongue may also be observed with bilateral supranuclear lesions in the course of pseudobulbar palsy.

## MOTOR SYSTEM

The routine examination of the motor system has been described in Chapter 1. As stated, evaluation of muscle bulk, power, and tone is essential, as well as a search for involuntary movements and appraisal of the

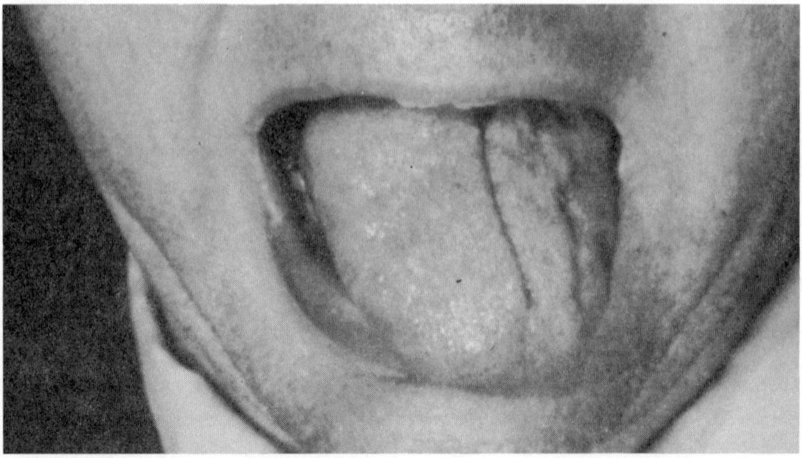

**FIGURE 2-21.** Infranuclear involvement of the left hypoglossal nerve in a patient with tumor of the glomus jugulare.

status of the muscle stretch reflexes. Additionally, cerebellar function must be assessed. Abnormalities may be found in any or all of these parameters of motor function in any given patient.

## Muscle Bulk

Changes in *muscle bulk* may be manifested as either atrophy or, less frequently, hypertrophy. *Atrophy* of muscles is most commonly encountered as the result of disease of the peripheral motor pathways, which comprise the anterior horn cell, peripheral nerve, and muscle (Fig. 2-22). It may on occasion result from cerebral involvement, probably as a reflection of disuse, but at times thought to reflect a trophic disturbance with parietal lobe affection. The distribution of atrophy is segmental in the case of anterior horn cell disease, or in the distribution of peripheral nerves in cases of involvement of these structures. In myopathies, atrophy is almost always symmetrical and proximal in distribution. When of cerebral origin, atrophy is often associated with a long standing hemiparesis and may involve both proximal and distal muscles in the affected limbs. In infantile hemiplegia, both muscles and bones of the affected side are smaller than those of the normal side, with resultant true hemiatrophy. The earlier the development of hemiparesis or hemiplegia in infancy, the more pronounced is the resultant asymmetry of somatic development.

The variety of atrophy occurring with parietal lesions requires special comment. The hand and arm tend to be more affected than the leg. The

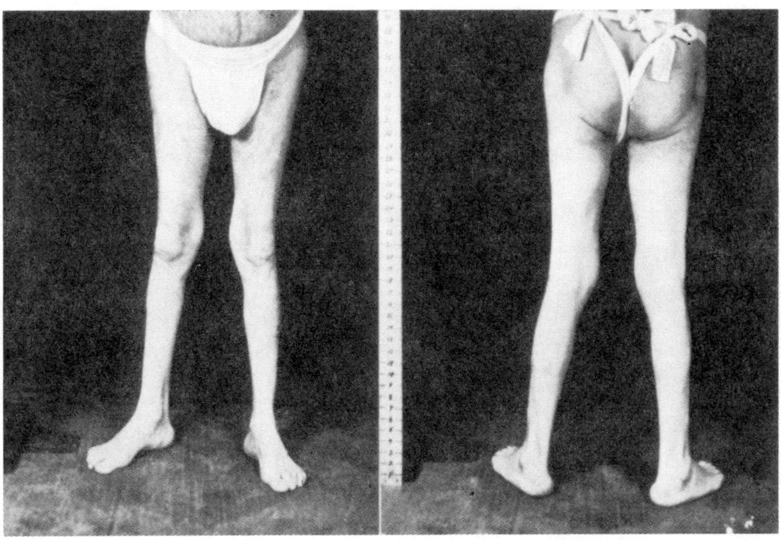

**FIGURE 2-22.** Atrophy involving the thigh and leg muscles due to poliomyelitis. Note the pas cavus from involvement of the intrinsic foot muscles.

atrophy of the small hand muscles may simulate closely that of peripheral denervation. The affected muscles are flabby and soft, the skin is thin, the fingers tapering, and there are trophic changes in the nails. The hands are often described as being effeminate in appearance. Hemiplegia or hemiparesis is usually but not invariably present, and varying degrees of sensory impairment are found, which involve particularly position sense. The explanation for the occurrence of atrophy under these circumstances is not known; as already indicated, it may reflect failure of some trophic influence originating in the parietal lobe, rather than simply disuse alone.

Segmental atrophy caused by cord disease may be difficult to map out precisely because of the tendency for muscles to be innervated from more than one segment. If the spinal cord disease is not diffuse, however, it may be possible to determine the segmental character of the atrophy, as in early cases of poliomyelitis with involvement of only a single muscle or a few muscles, or in the early development of amyotrophic lateral sclerosis, or syringomyelia, or cervical spondylosis with atrophy of only the small hand muscles. The pathogenesis of muscular atrophy in instances of denervation with anterior horn cell disease is not clear. It has been suggested that it, too, is the result of disuse, but it has also been thought that such atrophy may be the result of overactivity caused by repetitive muscle fasciculations (although drugs that increase fasciculatory activity seemingly have no effect on the rate of atrophy). Alternately, atrophy with anterior horn cell disease may result from the loss of tension engendered by the muscles now denervated.

Muscle atrophy is found in most diseases of the peripheral nerves. The degree and distribution of the atrophy depend on the extent of the injury to the nerve trunks. The presence of tenderness of the nerve trunks and of associated sensory alterations typical of most neuropathies should provide valuable assistance in distinguishing the atrophy of peripheral nerve disease from that caused by anterior horn cell involvement. Additionally, atrophy is found as a characteristic feature of virtually all intrinsic diseases of muscle (the myopathies), generally in a symmetrical and proximal distribution; on occasion, as in instances of myotonic dystrophy, atrophy may be predominantly distal. Finally, atrophy may be found in instances of arthritis in the muscles contiguous to the affected joints, as well as in muscles that have been immobilized for some time, as when encased in a cast.

There is no constant clinical pattern related to the rate of appearance of atrophy after partial or complete denervation. It may develop quickly or slowly and may be slight or pronounced. The factors determining such differences are not understood. In anterior horn cell disease, the degree of atrophy seems proportional to the number of motor units involved. Presumably the same holds true in peripheral nerve disease. Although the exact cause of muscle atrophy in primary disease of muscles is a matter of some dispute, it very likely is a reflection of the degeneration of isolated muscle fibers characteristic of most myopathies.

*Fasciculations* are irregular, fine or coarse twitchings of parts of muscles, which are generally not associated with movement of the affected limb. *Fibrillations,* which generally appear under much the same circumstances as fasciculations, are usually not visible through the skin, but are recorded electromyographically. Fasciculations tend to be associated with atrophy of muscles caused by denervation and appear particularly with disease of the anterior horn cells. They may be absent in atrophied muscles with advanced anterior horn cell disease, however, because there may be insufficient muscle remaining to exhibit this reaction. Conversely, they may appear early in anterior horn cell disease with little or no atrophy. There is thus no necessary or rigorous parallelism between the development of atrophy on the one hand and the appearance of fasciculations on the other. Often inconstant, fasciculations may be seen in muscles at one point in time, but not at another. They tend to appear at irregular intervals and shift in locus from muscle to muscle in a random manner. At times they are abundant and easily identified; at other times they may require careful search. Fasciculations are often intensified by exposure to cold. They may be elicited by mechanical stimulation of the muscle, for example, by sharply percussing a muscle or by placing the muscle in question on stretch. The administration of anticholinesterase agents may induce fasciculations as an unsought side effect; as an aid to diagnosis, such drugs may be used to intensify fasciculatory activity in patients with motor neuron disease.

Although commonly taken as indicators of anterior horn cell disease, it should be stressed that fasciculations are seen under other circumstances. Thus, they may be encountered in disease of the peripheral nerves, particularly when there is associated disease of the anterior roots and, presumably, retrograde changes in the anterior horn cells, as may occur in the Guillain-Barré syndrome (acute infectious polyradiculoneuropathy) and, at times, in diabetic or porphyric neuropathy. In addition, fasciculations appear commonly in anxious or fatigued individuals and may develop in instances of thyrotoxicosis. Fasciculations are also the primary manifestation of a disorder known as *benign myokymia,* or benign fasciculations, in which they appear repetitively in the same muscle or group of muscles for extended periods, often years, but without the development of atrophy, weakness, or reflex alteration, changes which might suggest the presence of anterior horn cell disease. Nonetheless, the predominant occurrence of fasciculations in anterior horn cell disease must be emphasized: once fasciculations are seen in the course of examination, diagnostic consideration must be given to such disorders as amyotrophic lateral sclerosis, progressive spinal muscular atrophy or other motor system diseases, syringomyelia, cord tumor, herniated disc, and other disorders in which the anterior horn cells themselves may be involved.

Muscle *hypertrophy* is perhaps most frequently encountered as a result of prolonged exercise in so-called *work hypertrophy;* a similar change is noted as a compensatory phenomenon in the face of weakness of other muscles. Muscular hypertrophy may also be found in association with some forms of congenital disease of the nervous system, perhaps particularly in cretinism, with or without associated involuntary movements, and in the rare occurrence of congenital hemihypertrophy, which involves one half of the body or of the face. A very rare disorder characterized by generalized muscular hypertrophy is known as *hypertrophia vera.* Muscular hypertrophy is also encountered in patients exhibiting myotonia; its occurrence under these circumstances is perhaps related to work hypertrophy. Enlargement of muscles may also be found in some forms of myopathy, particularly in the familial (sex-linked) progressive muscular dystrophy of childhood. Under these circumstances, the term *pseudohypertrophy* is more appropriately applied, since the enlarged muscles, commonly in the calves, have a rubbery consistency and are weak, in contrast to the normal or increased strength in true muscular hypertrophy.

## Muscle Tone

Changes of muscle tone must be searched for in all routine examinations. Increased muscle tone (spasticity or rigidity) or decrease or loss of muscle tone (hypotonia or flaccidity) may be observed. Interruption of the corticospinal pathway results in *spasticity,* characterized by an increase in muscle tone that is associated generally, although not necessarily, with increase in reflex activity and the appearance of pathologic reflexes, such as an extensor plantar response (Babinski sign). In spasticity there is an increase of resistance to passive movement, followed by a sudden release of resistance, generally referred to as a clasp-knife reaction. The presence of spasticity alone unfortunately gives no clue as to localization of the responsible lesion; it is indicative only of a lesion interrupting the corticospinal pathway at any point in its course, whether in the cerebral hemisphere, in the internal capsule, in the brainstem, or in the spinal cord. Generally speaking, the farther the lesion from the cortex, the more prominent is the spasticity. Interruption of the corticospinal pathway is, however, by no means invariably associated with spasticity. Particularly in acute cases, decreased muscle tone or flaccidity may appear initially as in so-called *spinal shock.* Flaccid paralysis caused by an acutely evolving lesion of the corticospinal system may last a few days to a few weeks and gradually gives way in the majority of instances to spasticity; on the other hand, flaccidity may persist throughout the course of the illness. The pathogenesis of spasticity is not entirely clear. It may very well reflect the end result of descending extrapyramidal, perhaps reticular, influences that act in unopposed fashion upon release from inhibitory control of the pyramidal system itself.

Disease of the extrapyramidal system, especially of the basal ganglia, results in a state of increased muscle tone referred to as *rigidity.* Rigid muscles demonstrate a plastic reaction, with an even, steady resistance to passive movement, which has been likened to the sensation of bending a lead pipe (hence the term "lead pipe rigidity"). At times the rigidity is intermittent and jerky, as in the cogwheel rigidity typical of parkinsonism.

*Hypotonia* or *flaccidity* is characteristic of affection of the lower motor neuron and is thus associated with disease of the anterior horn cells, spinal roots, or peripheral nerves. The muscles are loose and toneless; the affected limbs are hyperextensible and, at times, frankly flail-like. Hypotonia may also be encountered in disease of the posterior roots, presumably as a result of interruption of the afferent limb of the reflex arcs ordinarily operative in the maintenance of normal tone. Hypotonia is also typically found in cerebellar lesions, particularly with acute lesions, and appears to be a result of removal of cerebellar influence on descending brainstem and spinal reticular mechanisms.

## Muscle Power

Loss of muscle strength is invariably associated with disease of the upper or lower motor neuron or of the muscles. The degree of weakness tends to parallel the extent of injury of the structure concerned. When the weakness is partial it is referred to as *paresis,* when complete as *paralysis.* The term *hemiplegia* or *paraplegia* is applied to instances of complete paralysis of the affected limbs. The weakness of anterior horn cell or root disease is segmental in character and is associated with flaccidity, atrophy, fasciculations and loss of reflexes. That of peripheral nerve disease follows the distribution of the affected nerve or nerves and is thus predominantly distal in the common polyneuropathies; it is often associated with pain and sensory disturbances and is generally accompanied by loss of reflexes. The weakness of upper motor neuron disease is usually hemiplegic in character, tends to affect distal more than proximal muscles, is associated with spasticity, overactive reflexes and pathologic reflexes, and is without sensory change.

Not all weakness results directly from disease of the central or peripheral nervous system. Primary disease of muscle (i.e., myopathy) is invariably associated with weakness, almost always proximal in distribution. Marked weakness also results from interference with neuromuscular transmission, as in myasthenia gravis, curare poisoning, botulism, or in the Lambert-Eaton "myasthenic" syndrome of carcinoma of the lung. Transient paralysis occurs in electrolyte disorders, such as severe hypokalemia, and is characteristic of the periodic paralyses related to alterations of serum potassium levels; in these instances, interference with transmission of the electrotonic impulse along the sarcolemmal membrane by alteration of the normal ionic pattern is possibly the factor responsible for the clinical abnormalities.

Attacks of generalized muscular weakness that are induced by emotional excitement of any sort and at times result in complete although transitory collapse are found in the *cataplectic* episodes of narcolepsy. A number of patients so afflicted also wake from sleep on occasion to find themselves completely paralyzed for varying periods (so-called *sleep paralysis*). Both cataplexy and sleep paralysis are characterized by transient generalized loss of muscle tone and areflexia, features typical of the REM (rapid eye movement) stage of sleep; both have therefore been looked upon as representing fragmentary REM phenomena.

Loss of movement, it should be emphasized, is by no means necessarily indicative of paralysis *per se.* Profound impairment of movement often occurs with severe *sensory deprivation,* particularly loss of proprioception, without actual dysfunction of the motor apparatus itself. In such cases, the apparent weakness improves remarkably if the patient watches the limb during attempted movement. Loss or decrease of movement is also seen characteristically in paralysis agitans (Parkinson's disease), which is unassociated with weakness of any appreciable degree. This is noted in early cases as a loss of the normal arm swing, later in the course as loss of almost all voluntary movement. Patients with extrapyramidal diseases, such as parkinsonism, often do complain of weakness; this complaint ordinarily reflects not true weakness as such, but rather the slowness of movement and difficulty in initiating movements, that is, the bradykinetic and akinetic phenomena that are typical of such disorders. Loss of movement may also result from contractures, or from fixation of joints

**TABLE 2-3.** Synkinesis of upper extremity in pyramidal tract disease

| NAME | STIMULUS | RESPONSE |
|---|---|---|
| Wartenberg's sign | Active flexion of fingers about a stick | Flexion and opposition of thumb |
| Sign of Klippel and Feil | Passive extension of fingers (when there is some contracture in flexion) | Flexion and opposition of thumb |
| Souques' sign of interosseous muscles | Active elevation of extended arm | Extension and adduction of fingers |
| Strümpell's sign | Active flexion of elbow | Pronation and flexion of hand |
| Brachiobrachial synkinesis | Extension of flexed elbow of normal side by examiner against patient's resistance | Flexion of elbow on paralyzed side |
| Sterling's sign | Active adduction of shoulder on normal side against resistance by examiner | Adduction of shoulder on paretic side |

by trophic or other processes. Finally, impaired movement may be associated with catatonia and with hysteria. Under these circumstances, the nonanatomic distribution of weakness and the absence of associated atrophy or reflex changes are of substantial diagnostic import.

Accessory or synkinetic movements are seen under some circumstances, particularly in disease involving the corticospinal system (Table 2-3). Flexion movements of the fingers of a paralyzed hand may be observed in cases of hemiplegia when a patient squeezes the examiner's fingers with the normal hand. Dorsiflexion of the paretic foot in hemiplegia may be seen on flexion of the knee *(Strümpell phenomenon);* pronation of the paretic forearm may be found on extension of the arms upward *(pronator sign).* Awareness of such patterns of associated movements may be of help in achieving a correct diagnosis in patients with a hysterical paralysis. With true weakness of a leg, lifting the paralyzed leg while the patient is recumbent results in an increased downward pressure with the sound leg *(Hoover's sign),* which is perceived by the examiner with his hands placed under the patient's heels during the maneuver. In the hysterical patient, the downward pressure of the normal leg will be absent.

## Involuntary Movements

Involuntary muscular movements occur in a variety of forms and under many circumstances. Some, such as fasciculations, have been described above. Other patterns of movement disorders are as follows:

### TREMOR

Defined as involuntary, purposeless, and usually rhythmic movements of the limbs and, on occasion, of the head and trunk, tremor may be most simply approached on the basis of the circumstances under which the movements appear.

Tremor present when the limbs are in complete repose is referred to as a *resting tremor* and is characteristically encountered in instances of paralysis agitans (parkinsonism). The tremor here is rapid, affects particularly the distal muscles (forearms and hands), and often assumes a so-called pill-rolling quality. It may persist when the arms are held extended, sometimes with an increase in amplitude, but with volitional movement it customarily diminishes and returns to its original severity when the limb rests once again. A similar resting tremor may be encountered in hepatolenticular degeneration (Wilson's disease). In that condition, when the arms are held extended, a much more florid movement disorder also appears, which consists of coarse, irregular flapping movements often referred to as a wing-beating tremor, or flap. A similar but usually much finer flapping movement may be encountered in the metabolic encephalopathies, especially in severe hepatic or pulmonary disease; it tends to be particularly prominent in cases of impending hepatic coma. The term *asterixis* is sometimes applied to flapping movement of this sort; strictly speaking, asterixis is not truly a tremor in terms of a positive phenomenon of alternating movements of agonists and antagonists around a given joint but, rather, represents simply a transient but repetitive lapse of all postural tone.

A very rare form of resting tremor is encountered as a consequence of lesions involving the red nucleus. Referred to as a *rubral* tremor, this is an irregular movement at repose, waxing and waning in amplitude, at times disappearing completely, and frequently associated with intention tremor (see below).

In many conditions, tremor appears only when the arms are held extended in a *sustained posture* against gravity. Thus, a fine rapid tremor of the outstretched fingers is found in general paresis and is commonly associated with tremors of the tongue, eyelids, and lips. Fine tremors of the extended fingers and hands also appear in thyrotoxicosis, in conditions of fatigue or excitement, following the administration of agents such as epinephrine, amphetamine, or ephedrine, and in anxiety states. The use of cocaine, barbiturates, morphine, and bromides is often attended by similar movement; lithium may also result in a postural tremor of this sort, at times associated with resting tremor as well. A postural tremor may also follow exposure to industrial toxins such as metallic mercury. Tremors of the outstretched fingers commonly appear in the chronic alcoholic and may be very severe during periods of abstinence or withdrawal, as in the states of alcoholic tremulousness and delirium tremens; a curious inner sense of tremulousness often accompanies the somatic movements under these circumstances.

A coarse tremor of the outstretched fingers, sometimes increasing with voluntary activity, is the so-called *benign* or *essential tremor*. This involves males more than females and may make its appearance as early as adolescence. It is often inherited, usually as a dominant characteristic; when this is the case, the term *familial tremor* is applied. Sporadic instances tend to exhibit at a somewhat later age of onset than familial cases. In both varieties, the tremor initially involves the arms and may lead to considerable embarrassment as a result of spillage of food and drink. Eventually tremor of the head may appear and the voice characteristically becomes quavering. The movements are typically suppressed by alcohol; this may lead to excessive therapeutic utilization with resultant chronic alcoholism. This disorder is commonly misdiagnosed as paralysis agitans, despite the complete absence of other signs of extrapyramidal disease, as would be anticipated in the latter.

A coarse tremor of the fingers may be found in late life, generally in conjunction with a nodding or rotary tremor of the head, and is referred to as *senile tremor*. The movements may be present at rest, on movement, or with extension of the limbs. A tremor of the tongue may also be present.

Ordinarily there are no supplemental signs to suggest the presence of significant extrapyramidal disease.

Tremor, or more accurately tremulousness, may appear in a paretic limb during attempted movement. This is a nonrhythmic movement disorder that generally involves the proximal portion of the limbs particularly and is presumably due to faulty postural fixation of the weak limb.

Disease of the cerebellum or its pathways results in the appearance of an *intention tremor,* an oscillating, fairly regular tremor becoming evident on voluntary movement such as the finger-to-nose test; this tremor increases in amplitude in crescendo fashion as the goal is approached. Usually no tremor is evident at rest, but some movement may be visible when the arms are simply held in an extended manner. Intention tremor appears most prominently with affection of the superior cerebellar peduncle (brachium conjunctivum); it thus is observed most strikingly with softenings that result from occlusion of the superior cerebellar artery, or with any other lesion that implicates the dentatorubral pathway, for example, in multiple sclerosis.

## CHOREA

Choreic movements are quick, random, nonrhythmic movements of rather small amplitude, sometimes explosive in occurrence, involving both distal and proximal muscles. The hands are most frequently affected, and a constant play of twitching movements of the fingers may be seen. Patients so afflicted not uncommonly attempt to mask the nature of the choreic movement by converting the motion to a seemingly purposeful gesture. The trunk may be involved and the gait at times seriously disturbed. Facial grimacing and lip smacking and pursing movements are often encountered and may be difficult to distinguish from the orofacial dyskinesias characteristic of the disorder known as *tardive dyskinesia,* which appears as a result of the long-term use of phenothiazines and other dopamine antagonists. Some degree of muscular hypotonia commonly accompanies chorea, regardless of cause. Chorea characteristically occurs in Sydenham's (rheumatic) chorea, chorea gravidarum, and in Huntington's disease, but similar movements are occasionally seen under other circumstances, for example, following carbon monoxide poisoning ("symptomatic chorea"). In some of these disorders (e.g., Huntington's disease), significant lesions are observed in the striatum, particularly in the caudate, but under other circumstances a distinctive anatomic substrate cannot be identified. In the elderly, a similar movement disorder is referred to as *senile chorea.* On occasion, the movements of chorea may be extremely gross, capable of moving an entire limb in an irregular, abrupt flinging fashion (hemichorea); it may be very difficult to distinguish this from *hemiballismus,* a dramatic condition characterized by wild flinging or circling movements of the limbs tending to involve the arm more than the leg and most commonly associated with vascular lesions involving the subthalamic nucleus.

## ATHETOSIS

In contrast to the abrupt and predominantly distal movements of chorea, athetosis is characterized by somewhat slower snake-like movements, which involve distal muscles but with a tendency to spread proximally as well. Muscle tone is somewhat heightened as a rule. Athetosis may appear in many disorders affecting the basal ganglia. It is observed in infancy and childhood as so-called *double athetosis,* possibly reflecting birth hypoxia and associated pathologically with status marmoratus (marbled state, hypermyelinization) of the basal nuclear masses. Athetoid movements are seen in a variety of diseases characterized by a loss of proprioception in the involved limbs, such as subacute combined degeneration of the cord or tabes dorsalis; the term *pseudoathetosis* is applied here. Similar movements also may appear during recovery from hemiplegia *(posthemiplegic athetosis* or *chorea),* and under these circumstances impairment of proprioception is also commonly discerned. Choreiform or athetoid movements may occur on an episodic, intermittent basis in the rare disorder called *paroxysmal choreoathetosis.*

## DYSTONIA

This consists of slow writhing or twisting movements, which usually begin in the distal portions of the limbs but spread proximally to involve the girdle musculature as well as the muscles of the head, neck, and trunk. It reaches its most florid manifestation in that disorder known as *dystonia musculorum deformans.* Dystonia appears under many other circumstances, with both sporadic and familial occurrence, and is perhaps seen most commonly as an expression of an acute idiosyncratic response to the use of phenothiazines. Dystonic posturing may also be seen in a host of other movement disorders, for example, in cases of parkinsonism. As with chorea and athetosis, dystonia tends to be related primarily to dysfunction of the basal ganglia. In terms of speed of movement, distribution of movement, and muscle tone, it stands at the opposite end of the scale from chorea, with athetosis between. Fragmentary forms of dystonia are well recognized: thus, in *torticollis,* or *wry neck* (Fig. 2-23), the characteristic involuntary turning of the head and neck presumably reflects a partial or limited dystonic syndrome of uncertain etiology. *Writer's cramp* may similarly be looked upon as a fragmentary dystonic phenomenon.

## MYOCLONUS

Myoclonic movements are rapid, jerk-like contractions of either proximal or distal muscles, which are usually nonrhythmic but at times bilaterally symmetrical. They are encountered in a host of disorders. Myoclonic jerks may be seen in diseases characterized by extensive destruction of cortical

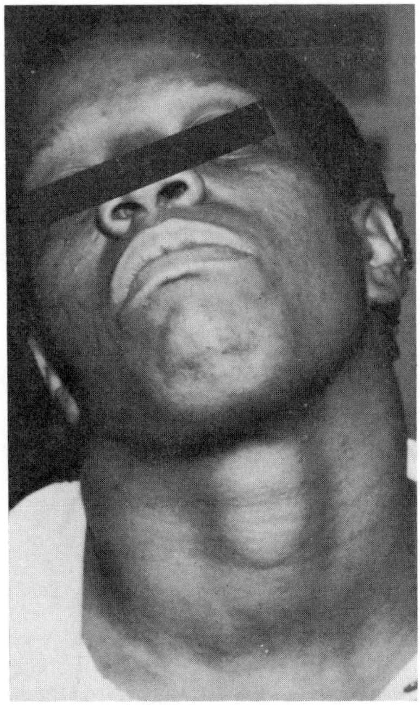

**FIGURE 2-23.** Spasmodic torticollis, demonstrating striking sternomastoid hypertrophy.

neurons, such as Tay-Sachs disease and Jakob-Creutzfeldt disease, as well as in inclusion body encephalitis with damage to both gray and white matter of the cerebrum. Encephalopathies that follow severe hypoxia and hypoglycemia may be accompanied by myoclonic jerks as well. Such movements are also an important feature of the so-called *myoclonic epilepsy of Unverricht,* in which major pathologic changes may be found in the cerebellar cortex or deep cerebellar nuclei. The rubric *hypnogogic myoclonus* is applied to brief, generally isolated myoclonic jerks that involve the entire body, or a limb or limbs, often noted by normal individuals when falling asleep or on arousal from sleep. Massive myoclonic jerks of the trunk *(salaam seizures)* appear in an uncommon infantile disorder known as *infantile spasms;* these movements are associated with a remarkably disorganized electroencephalographic pattern called hypsarrhythmia. The term *action myoclonus* (Lance-Adams syndrome) refers to sudden, brief, and often violent irregular myoclonic jerking of limbs that appears on attempted motion and is largely confined to the active limb(s); it is seen most frequently as a residual of severe anoxic encephalopathy.

Rapid, fluttering, rhythmic movements of the soft palate that are commonly associated with synchronous movements of the eyes, tongue, and jaw, are referred to as *palatal myoclonus* or *palatal nystagmus.* Not resembling myoclonus as seen under other circumstances, this disorder in the great majority of cases results from interruption, usually by softening, of the dentato-rubro-olivary system.

### SPASMS

A variety of spasms of the voluntary musculature are seen in neurologic disease. Habit spasms, commonly psychogenic in origin, may involve the face, limbs, or trunk. *Writer's cramp* consists of persistent, recurrent spasms of the musculature of the hand and has been variably interpreted as either a limited dystonic disorder or a hysterical manifestation that is encountered especially in certain occupational settings. Spasms of the tongue or of swallowing may be seen, which are again variously interpreted as being of psychogenic origin or caused by some form of basal ganglia disease. Spasms involving the somatic muscles commonly occur in patients with corticospinal tract disease; they are most often nocturnal in appearance and frequently painful. Extensive muscle spasms, precipitated especially by movement, are typical of the so-called *stiff man syndrome*. *Hemifacial spasm* is not uncommon; it may follow lesions of the facial nerve, or of the facial nucleus, but may also develop as a habit (psychogenic) spasm. *Blepharospasm,* consisting of spasmodic contractions of the eyelid, or eyelids, has been described following encephalitis, but is frequently encountered as a manifestation of anxiety.

### TICS

These may be defined as abrupt, asynchronous movements of the face, trunk, or limbs, which are at times difficult to distinguish from myoclonic jerks. Tics are often repetitive and stereotyped in appearance and are in the majority of cases psychogenic in origin. Remarkable compulsive tics are a hallmark of the syndrome of *Gilles de la Tourette,* whose pathogenesis remains obscure.

### SEIZURES

Although not ordinarily looked upon as movement disorders, seizures, particularly when focal, may at times be confused with the movement disorders already discussed. This is particularly true in instances of *epilepsia partialis continua*. A detailed discussion of epilepsy is, however, inappropriate at this juncture.

## Reflex Disturbances

### LOSS OF TENDON (MUSCLE STRETCH) REFLEXES

Loss of reflexes, or arreflexia, occurs most frequently in cases of interruption of the reflex arc, either on the efferent side, as in disease of the anterior horns, anterior roots, or peripheral nerve, or on the afferent side, as in affections of the posterior roots. The features that distinguish interruption of the reflex arc at its various levels are described in Chapter 3. Loss of reflexes may also occur in myopathy, usually in advanced stages of the disease and associated with muscle atrophy. The reflexes are lost temporarily during the episodes of paralysis of familial periodic paralysis, as well as in REM sleep and in cataplexy and sleep paralysis. In instances of spinal shock that result from acute transection or acute compression of the spinal cord, loss of reflexes is characteristically noted along with flaccid paralysis of the limbs. The stage of spinal shock may persist for 2 weeks to 2 or 3 months after the original injury; it may be replaced eventually by spasticity and overactive reflexes or, much less commonly, may persist indefinitely. Reflexes also disappear in comatose patients. Rarely, in apparently healthy individuals no patellar reflexes may be elicited; in some, all the reflexes may be hypoactive or absent entirely.

## INCREASE OR EXAGGERATION OF TENDON (MUSCLE STRETCH) REFLEXES

Increased reflex activity occurs in the vast majority of instances as a result of disease of the corticospinal (pyramidal) pathways. In such instances, the exaggerated reflexes are generally associated with abnormal reflexes such as the extensor plantar, and with spasticity, but not invariably so. In the presence of corticospinal disease, the superficial abdominal and cremasteric reflexes are commonly lost as well. As noted, synkinetic movements may also make an appearance in patients with corticospinal tract disease; these are summarized in Table 2-3. Overactive reflexes may also be found in extrapyramidal diseases such as paralysis agitans. Increase of reflexes is common in anxious subjects, but these reflexes are not pathologic. In patients with heightened reflexes, regardless of cause, spread of reflex activity is common.

## ABNORMAL REFLEXES (Tables 2-4 and 2-5)

**BABINSKI SIGN.** Associated with increased reflexes are various abnormal reflexes encountered with disease of the corticospinal system. Chief among these is the Babinski toe sign, which consists of extension of the great toe, usually with spreading (fanning) and flexion of the small toes, when the outer edge of the sole of the foot is stroked. It is probably better to refer to this sign as the *extensor plantar response,* since Babinski's name is actually applied to a number of other physical signs; traditionally, however, the term "Babinski sign" is applied to this reflex above all. This sign is virtually pathognomonic of corticospinal disease. It is never present in normal subjects except in infants during the first 6 months of life. While a Babinski sign may thus be taken as an indicator of disease of the corticospinal pathway, it is not invariably present under such circumstances, although other evidence of disease of this system may be abun-

**TABLE 2-4.** Pathologic reflexes of the lower extremity in pyramidal tract disease

| REFLEX | STIMULUS | RESPONSE |
|---|---|---|
| Babinski | Stroking outer edge of sole of foot | 1. Extension of great toe<br>2. Flexion of small toes<br>3. Spreading of small toes<br>4. Flexion of leg |
| Chaddock | Stroking lateral aspect of dorsum of foot and external malleolus | Extension of great toe |
| Oppenheim | Firm downward stroking of medial aspect of tibia | Extension of great toe |
| Rossolimo | Tapping balls of toes | Plantar flexion of toes |
| Mendel-Bechterew | Tapping dorsum of foot on outer surface | Plantar flexion of toes |

dant. Conversely, the Babinski sign may be the only evidence of corticospinal disease or the only residual of previous and more extensive disease. Care must be taken to avoid interpretation of a voluntary withdrawal extensor toe response as a Babinski sign. The toe extension in corticospinal disease is slow and usually disappears soon after the stimulus is removed; that of a voluntary response is faster and associated with rapid withdrawal of the leg. Transient extensor plantar responses may be found following generalized convulsions, in coma, and in many diffuse encephalopathies. At times, the plantar response is silent, rather than convincingly extensor; especially if unilateral, such a silent or immobile plantar response may have the same significance as a true extensor reaction.

None of the other signs that have been described in corticospinal tract disease appears with the same constancy as the Babinski sign. When present, they are looked upon as confirmatory evidence of disease. These include:

**OPPENHEIM'S SIGN.** Extension of the great toe on firm downward stroking along the medial side of the tibia.

**CHADDOCK'S SIGN.** Extension of the great toe on stroking the dorsum of the foot on its outer edge.

**GORDON'S SIGN.** Extension of the toe on firm compression of the calf.

**ROSSOLIMO'S SIGN.** Plantar flexion of the toes on tapping the balls of the toes. This sign is an unreliable indicator of pyramidal disease when

**TABLE 2-5.** Pathologic reflexes of the upper extremity in pyramidal tract disease

| NAME | STIMULUS | RESPONSE |
|---|---|---|
| Palm-chin reflex (Marinesco-Radiovici) | Stimulation of thenar region (median) | Contraction of muscles of chin and elevation of corner of mouth |
| Thumb-adductor reflex ("Babinski of the hand") Marie-Foix of the hand | Superficial stroking of hypothenar region (ulnar) | Adduction and flexion of thumb; sometimes flexion of adjacent digits and extension of little finger |
| Extension-adduction reflex (Dagnini) | Percussion of dorsum of hand (radial) | Slight adduction and extension of wrist |
| "Mendel-Bechterew of the hand" | Percussion of dorsal aspect of carpus and metacarpus (radial) | Flexion of fingers |
| "Rossolimo of the hand" | Percussion of palmar aspect of metacarpo-phalangeal joint | Flexion of fingers |
| Hoffmann's sign | Snapping nail of middle finger (median) | Flexion of thumb and fingers |
| Trömner's sign | Tapping palmar surface of tip of middle or index finger | Flexion of fingers and thumb |
| Gordon's sign | Compression of region of pisiform bone (ulnar) | Extension of flexed fingers |
| Chaddock's sign | Pressure of tendon of palmaris longus muscle | Flexion of wrist; extension of fingers |

found alone without a Babinski sign or evidence of weakness. In fact, it is normally found in children from 2 to 3 months to 2 to 3 years of age. A similar flexion of the toes is seen in *Mendel-Bechterew's sign,* which is elicited by tapping the dorsum of the foot on its outer surface over the cuboid bone; it is much less common than the Rossolimo sign.

**HOFFMAN'S SIGN.** Flexion and adduction movement of the thumb and flexion of the fingers when the terminal phalanx of the middle finger is lightly flicked, or when the nail of the middle finger is snapped. Although often said to be indicative of corticospinal disease, it connotes only a state of heightened reflex activity.

**TRÖMNER'S REFLEX.** Flexion of all the fingers including the thumb, as a modified finger flexor reflex. It is elicited as follows: The patient keeps his fingers flexed while the examiner taps with his middle finger the palmar surface of the tip of the middle or index finger of the patient. As with the Hoffman sign, this has been regarded erroneously as indicative of corticospinal disease, but implies only increased muscle tone of the fingers.

**FINGER-THUMB REFLEX (MAYER).** Opposition and adduction of the thumb combined with flexion at the metacarpophalangeal joint on firm passive flexion of the third to the fifth finger at the proximal joints. The reflex is positive in normal persons and absent in patients with corticospinal lesions. When lost on one side it may constitute a useful sign of a pyramidal tract lesion.

**WITHDRAWAL (FLEXOR) REFLEXES OF SPINAL AUTOMATISM.** After transection of the spinal cord, a state of spinal shock develops during which all reflex activity below the level of the lesion is lost. As recovery ensues, segmental reflex activity returns and is seen first as a return of flexion of the entire lower extremity. In transecting lesions of the spinal cord, these flexor reflexes are elicited by stimulating the skin of the trunk or limbs below the level of the lesion by pinching, pin-prick, scratching, application of cold, stroking the sole of the foot, or by the use of any noxious stimulus. The result is a massive reflex movement of flexion of the thigh and legs with dorsiflexion of the foot and toes. The movement is sometimes mistaken by the patient for a voluntary movement and as an indication of improvement. Physiologically this represents release of segmental flexor mechanisms from descending suprasegmental inhibitory influences. Such flexion reactions are seen most commonly in instances of complete interruption of the spinal cord by transection caused by injury, compression, or vascular disease. They may appear, however, without complete transection, but in the face of bilateral pyramidal tract disease, as in spastic paraplegia. The Babinski sign itself may be regarded as a fraction of a flexion reflex. In spastic paraplegia, stimulation of one leg will often result in flexion of this leg with crossed extension of the opposite limb. This is known as *Philippson's reflex.* A *mass reflex* may also be observed. This ensues on scratching or stimulating any part of the legs and consists of flexor spasms of the ventral abdominal wall and lower extremities, evacuation of the bladder, and sweating from an area of skin varying with the level of the lesion.

**POSTURAL REFLEXES.** These are much more evident in an experimental setting than in clinical practice. In decerebrate animals destruction of the labyrinths permits full exploration of the *tonic neck reflexes.* Thus, rotation of the head causes an increase in extensor tonus of the limb toward which the jaw points ("jaw limb") and relaxation of the limb toward which the vertex is rotated ("skull limb"). Flexion of the head toward one shoulder causes extension of the jaw limbs and relaxation of the skull limbs; extension of the head causes extension of the forelimbs and flexion of the hind limbs; and flexion of the head causes flexion of the forelimbs and extension of the hind limbs. Counterparts of these reflexes are seen in some situations in the human, particularly in infants up to 12 weeks of age, and in some cases of brainstem or bilateral corticospinal disease. Other postural reflexes, such as the Moro and lateral propping responses, are sometimes of importance in the evaluation of infants.

Of greater clinical significance, particularly in adults, is the *grasp reflex.* It is characterized by grasping movements in response to contacts felt in the palm of the hand, and reflex tonic grasping in response to stretching the flexor muscles of the fingers. The greater the stretch, the stronger the grasp. The grasp reflex is unaffected by loss of sensation of the skin of the hand or by visual stimuli, since it is found with undiminished intensity after local anesthesia of the hand and after blindfolding. It is regarded as a purely reflex phenomenon; care must be taken to exclude volitional activity. The grasp reflex and forced grasping have been found to indicate in general lesions of the opposite frontal lobe, but are normal occurrences in infants. The opposite of grasping, that is, *avoidance,* is sometimes encountered with parietal lesions.

**ADDITIONAL REFLEXES.** The *orbicularis oculi reflex,* elicited as already described, is diminished in facial palsies of peripheral origin, but preserved in central facial paresis. The *jaw reflex* is increased in bilateral supranuclear cerebral lesions. The *snout reflex,* brought out by tapping in the midline of the maxilla or mandible with a resultant rooting movement of the lips, is found in instances of diffuse cerebral dysfunction. The *sucking reflex,* consisting of involuntary pursing of the lips in response to visual or tactile stimuli, is normally present in infants. It appears in later life as a sign, either unilateral or bilateral, of frontal or diffuse cerebral damage. Like the grasp, it represents a return to a more primitive level of function.

Modes of elicitation of a number of other reflexes, and the segmental level of lesions responsible for their loss, are outlined in Tables 1-2 and 1-3.

## Disturbances of Station

Standing is a postural activity dependent on reflexes mediated through the medulla and influenced to a marked degree by tonic neck, labyrinthine, cerebellar, and proprioceptive mechanisms. Interference with any of the parameters responsible for the maintenance of local, segmental, or general static postural reflexes will cause impairment of the act of normal standing. Weakness or deformity of the legs will, of course, also interfere with the stance, though on an entirely different basis.

Disturbances of stance, or station, are characterized primarily by an inability to maintain normal equilibrium in standing, with the eyes either open or closed. As found in disease of the posterior roots or columns, such as tabes dorsalis, subacute combined degeneration, or Friedreich's ataxia, the difficulty is dependent on loss or impairment of deep sensation, which is manifested by a loss of position sense. Under these circumstances, *Romberg's sign* is positive; this is characterized classically by an inability to stand steadily with the feet together, the difficulty being increased with the eyes closed, that is, with removal of visual cues. A Romberg sign may be regarded as positive only if there is actual loss of balance during the maneuver, with a shift in the position of the feet in order to maintain equilibrium and prevent falling. Modest swaying of the trunk without loss of equilibrium should not be regarded as a positive Romberg sign.

If in early or mild cases Romberg's sign is not convincing, more definite difficulties may be brought out by asking the patient to maintain his balance on one leg alone with the eyes open or closed. This is ordinarily well performed by normal subjects but difficult or impossible for the patient with even mild disease of the posterior columns.

Disturbances of station are also found in diseases of the cerebellum or its pathways. In cases of cerebellar disease associated with truncal incoordination there is an inability to stand with the feet close together with the eyes either open or closed. Indeed, standing unsupported becomes impossible in advanced cases even with the legs widely separated. Traditionally, the disability in cerebellar disease, unlike that of posterior column disease, is not seriously affected by closing the eyes; however, removal of visual cues clearly increases truncal instability in some patients with pure cerebellar affection, despite normal proprioception.

Interference with standing is also found in disease of the labyrinth, or of the vestibular pathways, or in any disorder in which vertigo is prominent; in such instances it results from interference with spatial orientation and the false sense of motion that is associated with the sensation of vertigo. Patients with vertigo are unable to stand even with the legs widely separated, and they cannot walk a straight course.

## Disturbances of Gait

Impairment or loss of the normal act of walking is encountered in a wide variety of neurologic diseases. Normal locomotion is influenced by a number of bodily mechanisms and is the result of integration of many types of reflexes. It is dependent on simple reflex mechanisms at the spinal cord level, on righting reflexes maintaining the proper position of head, limbs, and trunk against gravity, on postural reflexes holding the body erect by maintaining extensor tone, and on neck and labyrinthine reflexes for regulating muscle tone and providing proper spatial orientation. It is also, of course, dependent upon normal strength and sensibility. Not surprisingly, therefore, the gait may be abnormal as the result of such diverse factors as loss of spinal cord reflex mechanisms, brainstem disorders, vestibular and cerebellar disturbances, proprioceptive loss, pyramidal tract disease, and cortical dysfunction. Certain typical forms of gait disorder require further discussion.

## STEPPAGE GAIT

Primarily a peripheral variety of gait alteration, the steppage gait is associated with foot drop and is seen in simplest form with a lesion of the external popliteal nerve itself or in its innervation from spinal segments L4-S1. The leg is flaccid and the gait characterized by foot drop with marked elevation of the thigh and leg in order to clear the dropped foot from the ground. The condition is sometimes bilateral, as in tumors involving the cauda equina or in bilateral involvement of the spinal cord in poliomyelitis. It is also bilateral in cases of peroneal muscular atrophy (Charcot-Marie-Tooth disease), and in advanced polyneuropathies of diverse cause.

Unilateral foot drop may be seen in sciatic neuropathy or in sciatica caused by a herniated intervertebral disc. In cases of sciatica, another form of gait disorder may also appear. In some such instances, the knee and hip are flexed on the painful side, the pelvis drops toward the painful side, and the gait is accomplished with short steps as the limb is flexed to avoid stretching the sciatic nerve.

A peculiar gait, also of peripheral origin and caused by pain, may be seen in cases of peripheral neuropathy (particularly of the "alcoholic" nutritional variety), in causalgias caused by nerve injuries, or in vasomotor disorders (erythromelalgia), all of which are associated with painful hyperesthesias and dysesthesias of the soles of the foot. In such cases weight-bearing is painful. The gait is with short steps, and limping and halting in character. The feet are commonly rotated so that the patient can avoid walking on the painful portions.

## WADDLING GAIT

This gait is seen in instances of muscular dystrophy, polymyositis, and other varieties of proximal muscular affection. It is characterized by a wide base, exaggerated lordosis, and a peculiar waddle with extension and lateral movement of the pelvis owing to weakness of the gluteal and truncal muscles.

## HYPOTONIC (TABETIC) GAIT

This gait abnormality, with hyperextension of the knees and loose, flail-like joints, is seen most characteristically in tabes dorsalis. The gait is broad based in an attempt to shift the center of gravity, the legs are lifted high in walking, the feet are slapped down firmly on the ground in order to elicit what proprioceptive reflexes may be available, and the eyes carefully watch the feet. The abnormality is greatly increased in the dark and with the eyes closed. A similar type of gait may be found in any disease involving the posterior column. At least superficially, this disability, which may be categorized at least in part as a *sensory ataxia,* resembles the ataxic gait of cerebellar disease.

## CEREBELLAR (ATAXIC) GAIT

This is characterized by inability of truncal, pelvic, and limb muscles to move in unison in a coordinated fashion. The patient walks with a widened base, the pelvis is held stiffly and tilted somewhat anteriorly, and the trunk and limbs are seemingly independent of the pelvis. The result is a disorganized gait with marked ataxia, the legs thrust forward from the hip in mechanical fashion without direction or coordination. Lurching and staggering are common. So incoordinate is the performance that patients with cerebellar disease are often accused of being intoxicated. Patients with this sort of gait abnormality generally have a lesion of the midline of the cerebellum, in particular, the superior vermis. In cases of midline cerebellar tumors and tumors that obstruct the fourth ventricle, the head may be held stiffly and anteriorly flexed, probably as a reflection of herniation of the cerebellar tonsils into and through the foramen magnum. A staggering, reeling ataxic gait is also encountered during acute vestibular disease, as in labyrinthitis, or in interruption of the vestibular pathways in the brainstem. Under such circumstances, the patient generally complains of *vertigo,* and associated signs of vestibular disease are found.

## SPASTIC GAIT

Disease of the corticospinal system is associated with gait disorders characterized primarily by spasticity. Chief among these is the *hemiplegic gait,* in which the arm is held spastically in a semiflexed adducted posture and the leg is spastic, extended, circumducted, and plantar flexed, a pattern so characteristic that it can hardly be misinterpreted. Bilateral disease of the corticospinal pathways results in a *spastic gait,* a shuffling type of gait with the legs stiff, extended, and scraping over the surface without being lifted from the ground. In some patients with a spastic gait, the legs, although spastic while attempting to walk, are actually quite limber on recumbency. In cerebral diplegia the severe spasticity of the legs produces a *scissors gait,* in which the legs cross over in front of one another as each is put forward; spasticity in these patients is usually associated with pronounced adductor hypertonicity.

## BASAL GANGLIA GAIT DISORDERS

Abnormalities of gait are seen in basal ganglia disorders, especially in *paralysis agitans.* In early cases only a loss of the normal associated automatic swinging of the arms is seen while walking; in advanced cases the head and body are flexed, the arms semiflexed and adducted in a posture reminiscent of a spastic attitude, the legs flexed and rigid, and the gait slow and shuffling *(marche à petits pas, festination).* Initiation of the act of walking is slow, so that there may be a long latency between arising from a chair and the beginning of the walking act. The gait is often propulsive, the patient walking with increasing rapidity as if chasing his own center of gravity; at times the reverse (i.e., a retropulsive gait) is seen. In *dystonia musculorum deformans* severe contortions give a ludicrous, bizarre appearance to the gait. In the various illnesses in which *chorea* is found, the sudden movements of the limbs or trunk may interfere with walking, at least in fleeting fashion; at times the gait has a lilting quality that resembles the movement of a skater.

## HYSTERICAL GAIT

Not easily described, the principal feature of a hysterical gait is its bizarre character; any type of performance may be encountered. *Astasia-abasia,* or complete inability to stand or walk with normal function of the legs when the patient is recumbent, may be seen in hysteria. It may also be encountered, however, with bilateral cerebral (particularly frontoparietal) disease as an expression of *gait apraxia* and may appear as a result of multiple vascular lesions, as in the so-called lacunar state with multi-infarct dementia.

# Disturbances of Coordination

The smooth coordination of muscular movement is impaired or lost under many different circumstances in diseases of the nervous system. Since normal coordination depends upon the proper functioning of agonists, antagonists, and synergists, it follows that any interference with the normal inter-relationships of these muscle groups will result in incoordination. *Weakness* of a muscle or limb will thus cause loss of coordination of movement because of muscular imbalance. A paretic arm consequently exhibits difficulty in performing smoothly the finger-nose test or rapid pronation and supination. Incoordination is also seen in the impairment of the finer movements of the thumb and fingers, particularly the index finger, in cases of disease of the corticospinal pathways. Fine movements, such as buttoning clothes and picking up small objects, are often lost.

Incoordination is also found in instances of interruption of the *posterior columns* or of the medial lemniscus. Under these circumstances, the incoordination is dependent on loss of proprioceptive impulses, is accompanied by loss of position or vibration sense, or both, and is increased on closing the eyes; it is commonly designated *sensory ataxia*. The ataxia of posterior column disease is characterized by dysmetria (i.e., errors in range of movement), with inability to measure distance properly, and resultant overshooting of the goal. Tremor may accompany the movement.

A special form of incoordination known as *asynergia* or *dyssynergia* is found in cerebellar disease. This is not dependent on disturbances of sensation and must be clearly distinguished from sensory ataxia (Table 2-6). It is characterized by dysmetria, by inability to perform movements smoothly (pronation-supination movements of the arms, rapid patting with the hands), and commonly by an associated disturbance of gait. Cerebellar dyssynergia may be mild or severe and may involve any or all parts of the body. Slight degrees of dyssynergia are brought out by the pronation-supination test; the patient is clumsy, his arm swings out more than normally, and he overpronates or supinates and loses the beat of the rhythmic movement of the test. In severe cases no rhythmic movement is

**TABLE 2-6.** Differentiation of cerebellar and posterior column incoordination

| | CEREBELLAR | POSTERIOR COLUMN |
|---|---|---|
| SENSORY DISTURBANCES | Absent | Always present: Loss or impairment of position and vibration senses |
| VISION | Symptoms variably increased by removing visual clues | Symptoms increased by obliteration of vision |
| DYSMETRIA | Reaches goal with intention tremor, or past-points with eyes open or closed | Past-points with eyes closed |
| TREMOR | On voluntary movement | Variable ("pseudo-athetosis") |
| GAIT | Wide-based, pelvis fixed, trunk and limbs moving asynchronously | Wide-based, steppage with eyes watching feet and ground |
| STATION | Romberg's sign not present, but unsteadiness in standing with eyes open or closed | Romberg's sign present |

possible. The cerebellar gait, which may be looked upon as an expression of dyssynergia of the trunk mucles, has already been described. It should be pointed out that the basic defect in all manifestations of incoordination in cerebellar disease may be one of faulty postural fixation, particularly at proximal joints.

Disease of the labyrinths, and of the vestibular nerve and the vestibular pathways in the brainstem, is also associated with incoordination characterized particularly by dysmetria, with past-pointing. The presence of nystagmus and especially of vertigo should assist in separating this from the deficit encountered in cerebellar disease.

## SENSATION

The methods of performing a sensory examination have been described in Chapter 1. The various patterns of altered sensibility consequent to lesions at the peripheral, radicular, spinal cord, brainstem, thalamic, and cortical levels will be discussed in Chapter 3.

## BIBLIOGRAPHY


Adams, R. D.,: *Diseases of Muscle.* ed. 3. Harper & Row, Hagerstown, Md., 1975.

Adie, W. J.: *Tonic pupils and absent tendon reflexes.* Brain 55:98, 1932.

Atkin, A., and Bender, M.: *"Lightning eye movements" (ocular myoclonus).* J. Neurol. Sci. 1:2, 1964.

Bender, M. B., and Strauss, I.: *Defects in visual fields of one eye only in patients with a lesion of one optic radiation.* Arch. Ophthalmol. 17: 765, 1937.

Black, P. M.: *Brain death.* N. Engl. J. Med. 299:338, 393, 1978.

Bowden, R. E. M.: *A comparative study of the rate of atrophy of skeletal muscle following anterior ramisection and acute anterior poliomyelitis in the rhesus monkey.* Bull. Hopkins Hosp. 89:153, 1951.

Bricola, A.: "Prolonged post-traumatic coma." In Vinken, P. J., and Bruyn, G. W. (eds.): *Handbook of Clinical Neurology.* vol. 24. American Elsevier Pub. Co., Inc., New York, 1976, p. 699.

Cogan, D. G.: *Neurology of the Ocular Muscles.* ed. 2. Charles C Thomas, Springfield, Ill., 1963.

Critchley, M.: *The Parietal Lobes.* Hafner Publishing Co., New York, 1966.

Darley, F. L., Aronson, A. E., and Brown, J. R.: *Differential diagnostic patterns of dysarthria.* J. Speech Hear. Res. 12:246, 1969.

DeJong, R. M.: *The Neurological Examination.* ed. 4. Harper & Row, New York, 1979.

Denny-Brown, D.: "The frontal lobes and their functions." In Feiling, A. (ed.): *Modern Trends in Neurology.* Butterworth & Co., Ltd., London, 1951.

Denny-Brown, D., and Chambers, R. A.: "The parietal lobe and behavior."

In *The Brain and Human Behavior.* vol. XXXVI. Proceedings of the Association for Research in Nervous and Mental Disease. Williams & Wilkins, Baltimore, 1958.

Fisher, C. M.: *Ocular bobbing.* Arch. Neurol. 11:543, 1964.

Glaser, J. S.: *Neuro-ophthalmology.* Harper & Row, Hagerstown, Md., 1978.

Harrington, D. O.: *The Visual Fields.* ed. 4. C. V. Mosby Co., St. Louis, 1976.

Lambert, E. H.: *Neurophysiological techniques useful in the study of neuromuscular disorders.* Assoc. Res. Nerv. Ment. Dis. Proc. 38:247, 1960.

Lance, J. W., and Adams, R. D.: *The syndrome of intention or action myoclonus as a sequel to hypoxic encephalopathy.* Brain 86:111, 1963.

Menkes, J. H.: *Textbook of Child Neurology.* Lea & Febiger, Philadelphia, 1974.

Nelson, J. R., and Johnston, C. H.: *Ocular bobbing.* Arch. Neurol. 22:348, 1970.

Plum, F., and Posner, J. B.: *Diagnosis of Stupor and Coma.* ed. 3. F. A. Davis Co., Philadelphia, 1980.

Schwab, R. S., Stafford-Clark, D., and Prichard, J. S.: *The clinical significance of fasciculations in voluntary muscle.* Br. Med. J. 2:209, 1951.

Smith, J. L., and Cogan, D. G.: *Optokinetic nystagmus in cerebral disease.* Neurology 10:127, 1960.

Traquair, H. M.: *An Introduction to Clinical Perimetry.* ed. 6. C. V. Mosby Co., St. Louis, 1949.

Uemura, T., et al.: *Neuro-otological Examination.* University Park Press, Baltimore, 1977.

Walsh, F. B., and Hoyt, W. F.: *Clinical Neuro-ophthalmology.* ed. 3. Williams & Wilkins, Baltimore, 1969.

Walshe, F. M. R., and Robertson, E. G.: *Observations upon the form and nature of the "grasping movements" and "tonic innervation" seen in certain cases of lesions of the frontal lobe.* Brain 56:40, 1933.

# 3

# TOPICAL DIAGNOSIS OF NERVOUS DISEASE

Neurologic diseases become intelligible only if a meaningful relationship can be established between the symptoms and signs on the one hand and a precise anatomic localization of the responsible lesion, or lesions, on the other. Localization of the disease process thus becomes the next logical step following the examination itself; in fact, if the locus of disease cannot be defined, its very nature may well escape clarification. The process of localization is an act of synthesis that follows rationally ordered steps that should be comprehensible not only to the skilled neurologist but to the student and generalist as well. Much material of importance in identifying the site of a lesion within the nervous system has been presented in the preceding chapter. Here, additional and supplemental material is provided in pursuit of this goal of establishing a topical diagnosis.

Although certain of the symptoms encountered in disease of the nervous system simply reflect loss of function as a direct consequence of a given lesion (e.g., paralysis with interruption of the motor pathway), many others are the expression not of the diseased or degenerated areas themselves, but of the activity of other portions of the brain or spinal cord, the action of which may emerge unopposed after the involved areas are rendered nonfunctional. It is essential to recognize the fact that destructive lesions, that is, those characterized by loss of parenchymatous elements, cannot produce positive symptoms. This was emphasized by Hughlings

Jackson, to whom belongs the credit for crystallizing this seemingly obvious principle. Thus, the spasticity and reflex changes found in hemiplegia cannot be the direct expression of an area of destruction within the internal capsule or in any portion of the corticospinal pathway *per se,* since it is obvious, in accordance with this principle, that a destroyed area cannot itself give rise to such positive phenomena. It follows, therefore, that many of the signs and symptoms found in patients with hemiplegia are actually the expression of activity of other portions of the neuraxis that are now acting in uninhibited fashion after the site of the lesion itself has been put out of action. Put another way, such clinical manifestations would appear to reflect release of lower centers from the control of higher centers. Thus, extrapyramidal manifestations of paralysis agitans, such as rigidity, tremor, and postural changes, cannot spring directly from loss of cells in the substantia nigra or basal ganglia as such, but must of necessity result from the uninhibited action of other parts of the nervous system that normally act in unison with the areas now diseased. Symptoms such as chorea or athetosis must be regarded in the same light. As another example of this principle, the signs of disease of the cerebellum probably result from the unopposed action of the cerebral cortex and brainstem, which are now released from the modulating influence of the cerebellum.

In brief, then, *positive* symptoms cannot be produced by *negative* lesions. The symptoms and signs manifest in any given patient at any point in time therefore represent a combination of symptoms of deficit, such as paralysis or sensory loss, along with symptoms of release, such as tremor, rigidity, or hyperreflexia. Understanding of this concept is basic to comprehension of the signs of disease of the nervous system in the broadest sense.

## DISTURBANCES OF INTEGRATIVE CEREBRAL FUNCTIONS

Lesions involving the cerebral hemispheres give rise to a number of abnormalities referable, for example, to motility, sensation, and vision, as will be described in detail below. Alterations in higher integrative function also appear. Some of these, such as changes in mentation, personality, or awareness of the body scheme, have been discussed in Chapter 2. There remain for consideration here those derangements of symbolic brain function generally referred to as aphasia, agnosia, and apraxia, identification of which is often of major importance in the delineation of hemispheral disease.

### Aphasia

Aphasia may be defined as a loss or impairment of language caused by a lesion or lesions that involve highly specific portions of the brain. In general, aphasias develop as a consequence of lesions in the dominant cerebral hemisphere, usually frontotemporal in location and particularly clustering about the insula (isle of Reil) (Fig. 3-1). In right-handed individuals the left hemisphere is dominant as regards localization of language function. The great majority of ambidextrous and left-handed individuals also exhibit a dominant left hemisphere, although in these patients dominance is commonly less clear-cut than in right-handed individuals. Occasionally, definite right hemispheral dominance is evident. It is not always possible to determine with assurance which hemisphere is dominant on clinical grounds alone; in fact, traditionally dominance has often been determined after the fact by resorting to detailed neuropathologic evaluation in selected cases. If it is essential to determine hemispheral dominance during life, the intracarotid administration of sodium amytal is often used (Wada-Rasmussen test). Since such a carotid injection is not without hazard, attempts have been made to utilize noninvasive procedures. Dichotic listening has been utilized for this purpose in recent years but unfortunately lacks the required reliability.

Aphasia clearly has great localizing value in neurologic diagnosis. If care is taken in examination its presence can ordinarily be detected fairly readily, and its principle subgroups identified with reasonable accuracy.

Aphasia is a true disorder of symbolic language and must be distinguished from *dysarthria,* which consists of indistinctness in enunciation of words caused by interference with the peripheral speech mechanism (pharynx, larynx, tongue). As described in Chapter 2, dysarthria is observed in bulbar paralysis with nasal speech reflecting palatal immobility; as indistinctness of speech owing to weakness or paralysis of the

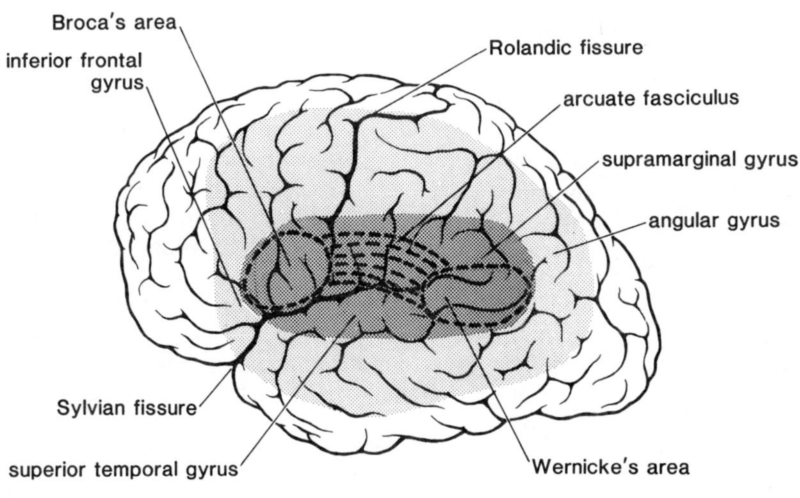


**FIGURE 3-1.** Portions of the left cerebral hemisphere considered most important in the development of aphasia in a right-handed individual. Perisylvian and border-zone areas are distinguished by intensity of shading.

tongue in patients with hemiplegia or motor system disease; as indistinct, muffled speech in extrapyramidal disorders such as paralysis agitans or hepatolenticular degeneration; as slurring or scanning and poorly modulated speech in patients with disease of the cerebellum; and in a host of other circumstances. Both aphasia and dysarthria must in turn be distinguished from *speech apraxia,* a disorder of speech expression in which the peripheral motor units of speech are intact (unlike dysarthria), but in which the speech mechanisms cannot be used in a coordinated fashion to articulate meaningful phonemes, words, or phrases; this could be likened to an "executive" disorder of verbal expression. In contrast to the situation in aphasia, symbolic language is preserved, as evidenced by the ability to read and write and by the absence of a disorder of receptive language. This variety of expressive disorder is generally encountered with lesions that involve the posterior portion of the dominant inferior frontal convolution and probably accounts for at least some instances of so-called pure expressive aphasia.

A sound vocal apparatus is necessary for the normal development and production of speech. Equally essential is a normal receptive mechanism (related to both auditory and visual perception). In the acquisition of speech during infancy and childhood, kinesthetic and auditory cues (playback) seem to play particularly critical roles; the importance of the latter is especially evident in the speech disorders of the child deaf from birth or an early age. Disorders of these perceptual functions, or isolation (disconnection) of those parts of the brain responsible for such perceptual functions from the perisylvian language areas, may play an important role in the production of aphasia in any age group.

## TESTS FOR APHASIA

Although severe disorders of language can be readily recognized, accurate diagnosis of more subtle aphasic disturbances requires careful testing at the bedside. A relatively small number of carefully chosen tests, when properly applied, will supply much valuable information in this regard (Table 3-1). Hastily and haphazardly applied testing, on the other hand, yields only fragmentary and often misleading data, of limited value at best. In the course of such testing, the patient with a language disorder may become depressed, agitated, and disturbed and will often refuse to cooperate further with the examiner. This response has been called a *catastrophic reaction* (Goldstein) and may reflect the patient's increasing awareness of the depths of his disability under the pressure of direct evaluation and observation.

Appropriate bedside testing of language function should include the following:

**SPONTANEOUS SPEECH.** If the aphasic patient can be made to speak, the spontaneous speech utterances will often provide most valuable in-

**TABLE 3-1.** Evaluation of the patient with aphasia

1. Determination of handedness (cerebral dominance)
2. Spontaneous speech
   - Enunciation
   - Fluency
   - Rhythm
   - Melody
   - Grammar
   - Word substitutions
   - Perseveration
   - Hand and facial gestures
3. Repetition
4. Naming
5. Comprehension of verbal symbols (auditory receptive tests)
   - Response to verbal commands
     - Single stage
     - Multistage
6. Comprehension of written symbols (visual receptive tests)
   - Recognition and comprehension
     - Letters
     - Words
     - Phrases
     - Sentences
   - Recognition of nonverbal images
7. Writing
   - Automatic (name, address)
   - Spontaneous
   - To dictation
8. Response of patient to testing

formation. Indeed, meticulous attention to spontaneous speech may prove as informative as the performance of formal language testing. Hesitancies and gaps in the normal flow of speech, syntactical errors, misuse of words, substitutions of words (paraphrasias, neologisms), and the appearance of a so-called word salad are all examples of the abnormalities that may appear during spontaneous speech. Perseveration is common in the aphasic, and disorders of rhythm and melody (dysprosody) may accompany the language disorder. In patients who are capable of understanding what is requested of them, the ability to name common objects and to repeat words and sentences should also be explored.

Assessment of the degree of *fluency* is often of substantial benefit in categorizing the nature of the language disorder as well. Thus, some aphasics will speak easily, often with a normal rate, rhythm, and melody; in general, patients who exhibit such fluency are found to have lesions in the more posterior (i.e., parietotemporal) language areas. In contrast, it may be difficult or indeed impossible to get an aphasic patient to speak spontaneously. Nonfluency of this type tends to be related particularly to more anteriorly placed lesions, as is the case with the predominantly expressive aphasic who is reluctant to speak, or incapable of doing so, because he lacks words. These distinctions are not entirely rigid; thus, a patient with an auditory receptive (i.e., posterior) aphasia may actually appear nonfluent because he is unable to understand requests to speak. Despite difficulties of this sort, an attempt should be made to categorize aphasia on this basis, and persistence on the part of the examiner will yield rich dividends.

**AUDITORY RECEPTIVE TESTS.** The understanding of the spoken word can be evaluated by two relatively simple tests:

1. By requesting the patient to follow simple commands ("put out your tongue," "close your eyes"), gradually increasing the complexity of the command until the patient is dealing with two or more orders ("close your eyes and open your mouth," "open your mouth, raise your hand, and close one hand," etc.). Some aphasics exhibit difficulty particularly when requested to cross the midline; thus, a request to touch the right ear with the left hand should always be included in testing of this sort.
2. By lining up a number of objects that can be produced from a pocket (matches, coin, key, etc.) and with specific commands determining whether the patient understands what is requested ("show me the key," "show me the coin," etc.).

**VISUAL RECEPTIVE TESTS.** These can be carried out at the bedside by asking the patient to read from a paper or a magazine and to interpret what has been read or by requesting him to follow a few simple written commands. The patient should be asked to read both aloud and to himself. It should be noted whether there is loss of the ability to read words or whether there is only mispronunciation of the words read. If the capacity to read is lost (alexia), it should be noted whether there is loss of recognition of letters or words, and whether the understanding of words as symbols is impaired or lost. The ability to recognize other visual images, for example, pictures of common objects, must also be tested.

**WRITING TESTS.** These are performed simply by asking the patient to write a spontaneous thought and also to write to dictation. The ability to write one's name is in itself a virtually automatic act and probably insufficient if not actually misleading when utilized as a sole criterion of the patient's ability to write. Obviously the patient with a hemiplegia that involves the dominant hand cannot be expected to write with that limb; the nonpreferred hand may be used in such a patient.

More extensive and elaborate tests may of course be undertaken and are particularly essential for investigative purposes; for routine bedside purposes, however, the aforementioned modes of evaluation will prove ample for the aphasic patient.

## CLASSIFICATION OF APHASIAS

A number of classifications of disorders of language have been suggested over the years; all are subject to criticism, in part because it is difficult to achieve a classification that is all-inclusive, and in part because any classification tends to create strict and perhaps artificial categories. Some such classifications are based on the clinical characteristics of the disorder(s), while others are based on the anatomic distribution of lesions responsible for the defect, where these can be identified with precision; yet others combine these approaches. Among the classifications based upon the *clinical characteristics of the language dysfunction,* one widely applied scheme is based on the volumetric, quantitative production of speech, that is, on the basis of fluency (Geschwind). *Fluent* aphasias are exemplified by speech that is produced effortlessly and with good articulation, grammar, rhythm, and prosody, but that is often meaningless and devoid of content. Words are used incorrectly, and paraphrasia is commonplace. *Nonfluent* aphasia, on the other hand, involves a very restricted speech output, which is generally associated with poor articulation in a simplistic, telegraphic style.

The fluent aphasias include:

*Wernicke's (receptive) aphasia,* which is characterized by inability to understand or repeat verbal symbols and caused by a lesion in the dominant superior temporal region posteriorly (Wernicke's area).

*Conduction aphasia,* with loss of the ability to repeat words but with preservation of language comprehension, which is due to a lesion in the suprasylvian parietal white matter (parietal operculum, arcuate fasciculus), a lesion that effectively disconnects the receptive from the motor speech areas.

*Amnesic (anomic) aphasia,* with preservation of powers of both understanding and repetition but difficulty in use of nouns (nominal or substantive words), which is commonly due to a focal lesion in the angular gyrus.

*Transcortical aphasia* which is due to isolation of the parasylvian speech area from other parts of the cortex and characterized by preservation of powers of repetition but with loss of comprehension.

The nonfluent aphasias include:

*Broca's (expressive) aphasia,* with a lesion in the posterior portion of the inferior frontal convolution (Broca's area).

*Global aphasia* which comprises a severe disorder of both expression and comprehension and is associated generally with destruction of both Broca's and Wernicke's areas.

An example of a classification based on the *anatomic distribution of responsible lesions* is that posited by Benson, as follows:

- Perisylvian Aphasic Syndromes
  - Broca's (expressive) aphasia
  - Wernicke's (sensory) aphasia
  - Conduction aphasia
- Borderzone Aphasic Syndromes
  - Transcortical motor aphasia
  - Transcortical sensory aphasia
  - Mixed transcortical aphasia
- Subcortical Aphasic Syndromes
  - Thalamic aphasia
  - Striatal aphasia
  - Aphasia of Marie's quadralateral space
- Nonlocalizing Aphasic Syndromes
  - Anomic aphasia
  - Global aphasia

Yet other classifications are based on clinical features, such as the preservation of powers of repetition or on linguistic criteria; the latter is detailed below. In any case, the plethora of classification schemes itself suggests the unsatisfactory nature of any one plan of categorization. Herein, disorders of language are presented on the basis of relative clinical significánce, without adherence to any single rigid scheme. Although such an approach may lack the appearance of cohesion, it has utility for the student and non-neurologist who are attempting to cope with such problems at the bedside. The salient features are summarized in Table 3-2.

At the outset, it must be emphasized that the various forms of language disorder detailed here, such as expressive (motor) aphasia or receptive (sensory) aphasia, refer only to the most dominant aspect of speech that is affected in any given individual. *It is extremely rare to find a pure form of language disturbance.* Hence, an expressive aphasia is characterized by predominantly expressive deficits, but a defect in comprehension is almost always present. The reverse is true for receptive aphasia. At times, the predominance of one form of aphasic utterance overshadows only slightly the other affected form. On occasion, as in so-called visual-receptive aphasia, a pure or almost pure form of deficit can be recognized. In all aphasic patients, the extent and severity of the deficit at any given point in time reflects a number of nonspecific factors, such as the patient's mood, interest, familiarity with the test situation, degree of fatigue, length of attention span, and presence and severity of mental confusion. Inconsistency of response is a characteristic feature of many aphasics and reflects to a greater or lesser degree factors such as these.

**TABLE 3-2.** Comparison of major forms of aphasia

| | EXPRESSION | VERBAL COMPREHENSION | REPETITION | NAMING | READING COMPREHENSION | WRITING | LESION |
|---|---|---|---|---|---|---|---|
| EXPRESSIVE (Broca's) | Nonfluent | Rel. intact | Impaired | Impaired | Variable | Impaired | Posterior-inferior frontal (Broca's area) |
| RECEPTIVE (Wernicke's) | Fluent | Impaired | Impaired | Impaired | Impaired | Impaired | Posterior-superior temporal (Wernicke's area) |
| GLOBAL | Nonfluent | Impaired | Impaired | Impaired | Impaired | Impaired | Frontotemporal |
| CONDUCTION | Fluent | Rel. intact | Impaired | Impaired | Variable | Impaired | Arcuate fasciculus; supramarginal gyrus |
| NOMINAL | Fluent | Rel. intact | Intact | Impaired | Variable | Variable | Angular gyrus; posterior-superior temporal |
| TRANSCORTICAL MOTOR | Nonfluent | Rel. intact | Intact | Impaired | Variable | Impaired | Anterior perisylvian |
| TRANSCORTICAL SENSORY | Fluent | Impaired | Intact | Impaired | Impaired | Impaired | Posterior perisylvian |

## EXPRESSIVE (MOTOR) APHASIA (BROCA'S APHASIA)

This language disorder is characterized by loss or impairment of the ability to express oneself and varies in degree from minor difficulty in finding words to virtually complete loss of all speech, that is, mutism. It comprises a defect in language ideation and formulation, in contrast to speech apraxia, in which the disorder is one of motility of the speech apparatus, and in which the symbolic functions of language are preserved. *Orofacial apraxia,* which is defined as an inability to utilize the muscles of the face, tongue, and articulatory apparatus in a coordinated manner, is, however, commonly encountered in patients with expressive aphasia. Patients with this form of aphasia demonstrate the following clinical features:

**INABILITY TO FIND WORDS.** The inability to find words with which to express thoughts may consist simply of occasional loss of a word, as evidenced by hesitations in speech. In such instances, the lapse may never be filled with the proper word and the patient may either pass on after great effort to express himself or burst into tears or profanity because of the inability to express himself; alternately, the patient may substitute another word that obviously has no connection with what he is trying to say, but which may sound somewhat like the desired word. In more advanced cases, words are lost in profusion, and the patient is unable to find the name of familiar objects and persons. Retardation in the rate of verbalization is striking; a lack of fluency is thus highly characteristic. *Dysprosody* is often encountered, in which the patient speaks monotonously with little or no inflection and without the normal melodic and rhythmic qualities of spoken language. Mispronunciations are frequent; defective articulation with frank slurring may appear. As a rule, the expressive aphasic recognizes his own errors and attempts to make amends by casting about for the correct word or words. In so doing, he may attempt to form words that sound like those he is seeking (paraphrasia) and for this reason may create unintelligible words. He may, for example, simply substitute one letter for another (e.g., "hatch" for "catch," "boat" for "coat"). In addition to substitutions such as these, which are based primarily on phonemic similarities, replacements may also be based on word associations (e.g., "table" for "chair," "spoon" for "fork"). Characteristically, the expressive aphasic evidences difficulties in the grammatical construction of language and may employ only nouns and verbs, using only an occasional adjective or adverb; this feature, coupled with the tendency to leave out words that cannot be found, results in a telegraphic style of communication with remarkable simplification of sentence structure. Word order reversals may also appear, and words may be used erroneously. Perseveration is common, and repetition is often impaired. In brief, the language of the expressive aphasic is characterized by frequent hesitations in speech with reduced fluency and with a loss of words which results in simplification and breaks in the continuity of expression.

Even in patients with severely restricted language output, automatic word series may at times be evoked with remarkably little difficulty, in the form of such automatic responses as rote recitations (e.g., alphabet, nursery rhymes). Some patients may be able to sing such rote series or rhymes, although they are unable to recite them without the aid of music. The automatic phraseology of social intercourse (e.g., respones to greetings of "Good morning") may also be preserved.

The phenomenon of *retained utterances* requires clarification. This abnormality is especially noteworthy in patients with expressive aphasia. It takes the form of automatic or emotional responses, at times cursing, which are commonly repeated in stereotyped fashion, appear unpredictably, and in some severely affected patients comprise the entirety of spoken language. The phrases uttered are often clearly articulated and at times explosive in quality. They may appear at appropriate times, as during attempts at verbalization, or may emerge inappropriately with no obvious external stimulus. Whether these utterances truly reflect a preserved island of language, or whether in at least some patients they actually represent simply expressions of extreme frustration, remains a matter of conjecture.

It is commonly held that individuals who are multilingual tend to lose the more recently acquired tongue when aphasia develops, that they revert thus to their natural speech, although with varying degrees of fluency. This statement probably requires some modification: careful study suggests that in the multilingual patient aphasia develops to an equal degree in all languages equally known, that is, languages equally known are equally lost. The examiner's own lack of facility in the native language of such patients may contribute to misinterpretation in this regard.

**DIFFICULTY IN WRITING (DYSGRAPHIA).** Writing is language recorded on paper; hence the expressive aphasic generally shows the same disability in his writing as in his speech. The defect ranges from occasional loss of words to complete inability to express himself. Calligraphic, spelling, and grammatical errors may all be encountered, even when the patient attempts to use the left (nonpreferred, nondominant) hand for writing in the face of a right hemiparesis.

**RETENTION OF UNDERSTANDING.** The patient with expressive aphasia commonly understands both the spoken and written word in a broad sense, although at least subtle impairment of comprehension is ordinarily encountered if sought. Thus, if examined carefully, the patient with an expressive aphasia will virtually always demonstrate auditory receptive dysphasic elements that are characterized by difficulty in understanding what is said to him. This may be evident only when complex commands are given. Reading comprehension is usually preserved, but reading aloud is difficult, paralleling the problem with spontaneous speech. As already indicated, these associated disorders of symbolic language permit differentiation of a true expressive aphasia from a speech apraxia.

Expressive aphasia is most commonly the result of a lesion in the posterior portion of the third (inferior) frontal convolution (Broca's area) in the dominant, and thus usually left, hemisphere. In the great majority of cases, the responsible lesion involves not only cortex but deep subcortical structures as well; the larger the lesion, the more severe is the disorder of language.

## RECEPTIVE (SENSORY) APHASIA (WERNICKE'S APHASIA)

In this type of dysphasia a disturbance or loss of the comprehension of speech predominates; the patient finds it difficult or impossible to understand the spoken and often the written word. The degree of deficit depends on the extent of destruction of the area affected and varies from only slight or moderate loss of understanding of words by ear to virtually total lack of comprehension in which the patient fails to respond at all to verbal stimuli. Even in severe cases fragmentary comprehension may be observed at times. In some patients, words are understood only in a very restricted fashion with an inability to appreciate their full significance, and responses tend to be concrete and simplistic. It should be noted that patients with a receptive aphasia commonly understand what may be called whole-body commands, for example, "stand up," or "turn around," while exhibiting severe difficulty in comprehension of other commands (which thus suggests a possible role of the nondominant hemisphere in whole-body functions). The receptive aphasic ordinarily exhibits severe impairment of repetition; however, the rhythm, melody, and articulation of speech are all normal. It should be stressed that the patient with receptive aphasia is capable of hearing sounds and words adequately; the defect is one of comprehension, in terms of what might be called *word deafness.* The patient who in contrast fails to respond to *all* auditory stimuli is either deaf or suffering from a true auditory agnosia. Involvement of visual language typically accompanies receptive aphasia. Referred to as *dyslexia* or *alexia,* this varies considerably in extent from patient to patient.

Disturbances in *expression* of varying severity are commonly encountered in the patient with a receptive aphasia. One may observe incorrect grammatical constructions, the wrong use of words, and substitutions of words and even whole phrases in a meaningless jumble. The expressive aphasic, when at a loss for a word, hesitates and fails to produce it, and is, thus, nonfluent. The receptive aphasic, on the other hand, simply substitutes another word and proceeds as if nothing were awry, with no attempt at self-correction; he thus exhibits a fluid, albeit abnormal, pattern of verbalization, which amounts at times to a true pressure of speech, or *logorrhea.* Unlike the expressive aphasic, the person with a receptive aphasia is unaware of his errors, largely because of his lack of understanding of auditory impressions, that is, his lack of the ability to monitor his own (and others') speech. Paraphrasia, grammatical confusions, and syntactical errors are typically found and neologisms may be prominent. Verbal confusions are frequent. Verbal substitutions occur, and whole phrases may be inserted in the speech in erroneous fashion. As a result, the speech production in severe cases of receptive aphasia is likely to be a disjointed and unintelligible hash or *word salad;* the term *jargon aphasia* is often applied to this state of affairs. *Difficulties in writing* (agraphia) under these circumstances may be as great as those of speech and are of a similar order; like speech, writing is inclined to be profuse but confused.

In *visual receptive aphasia,* that is, *alexia* or word blindness, there is loss of understanding of the printed word and failure to comprehend words as symbols. In patients so afflicted, the capacity to identify letters may be retained, but their synthesis into, and meaning as, words is lost. At times even individual letters fail to be recognized. In defects of a minor degree there may be recognition of some or most of the words in a sentence, but inability to synthesize the meaning of the sentence itself. Alexia commonly appears in association with homonymous hemianopsia and with disorders of both written and spoken language. It may appear as part of the syndrome of *visual object agnosia,* in which not only written symbols but all manner of objects fail to be identified by visual clues alone. Rarely, alexia, or *pure word blindness,* is encountered in isolation, without other disturbances of symbolic language, either spoken or written (often referred to as the syndrome of alexia without agraphia). An inability to recognize colors, *color agnosia,* may accompany the reading deficit. In some patients, a curious difference may be noted in the degree of disability as regards reading of letters or words on the one hand and reading of numbers on the other.

Of considerable interest in the context of alexia is that condition known as *congenital word blindness* or *developmental dyslexia.* Although of a different order from acquired dyslexia, this inborn and sometimes familial defect may be of great importance in instances of delayed or imperfect acquisition of reading skills in the young. It appears to be a significant although probably uncommon cause of learning disability in the intelligent child without brain damage. A disorder of writing and spatial conceptual defects are sometimes found as associated abnormalities in the dyslexic child.

Receptive aphasia results in the majority of cases from a lesion in the posterior portion of the first (superior) temporal convolution in the dominant hemisphere. The lesion responsible for alexia accompanied by agraphia tends to be more posteriorly placed and involves the dominant angular gyrus. Lesions in the splenium of the corpus collosum and in the left visual cortex appear to be critical in the production of the syndrome of pure alexia without agraphia. The anatomic substrate of developmental dyslexia is not known.

## EXPRESSIVE-RECEPTIVE APHASIA (MIXED OR GLOBAL APHASIA)

Patients with this form of language disorder characteristically exhibit a severe loss of both expressive and receptive elements of language. The expressive loss is usually so great that only a few sounds or words remain and the capacity to make even simple sentences is lost. Retained utterances may appear, but the use of automatic phrases is commonly inappropriate, and true propositional language is lacking. Understanding of words is greatly limited; the patient often fails to understand even single words or simple phrases. Repetition, naming, reading, and writing are all impaired. Generally such patients exhibit an extensive neurologic deficit in addition to the disorder of language. Although the clinical course is variable, many patients with global aphasia improve and ultimately demonstrate one or other of the more restricted aphasic syndromes.

The precise location of the lesion responsible for global aphasia cannot be identified with certainty. Extensive destructive lesions that involve the language area of the dominant hemisphere are generally noted.

## CONDUCTION APHASIA

This form of language disorder not uncommonly emerges during recovery from a severe receptive (Wernicke's) aphasia. It is a fluent language disorder that is characterized by severe impairment of repetition, difficulty in reading aloud (but with good reading comprehension), disturbance of writing, and marked paraphrasia, but generally with well-preserved comprehension of spoken language. Many patients so afflicted exhibit a right hemiparesis with or without cortical sensory loss and, at times, a curious pain syndrome reminiscent of the thalamic syndrome (see p. 156). Pain asymbolia (failure to appreciate painful stimuli) has been noted in some. Hemianopic field defects are common. Orofacial and limb apraxia are frequent and often severe; the latter involves both arms. Anomia is severe.

A lesion that interrupts intrahemispheral associational systems, specifically the internal arcuate fasciculus in the parietal operculum, has been most often implicated in causation of this disorder. The arcuate fasciculus connects Wernicke's area in the superior temporal gyrus with Broca's area in the frontal operculum; thus, disconnection of Wernicke's from Broca's area is thought to account for the clinical manifestations of this disorder. Involvement of the supramarginal gyrus has been implicated in some patients.

## AMNESIC (NOMINAL) APHASIA (ANOMIA, DYSNOMIA)

Although difficulty in naming is found in virtually all disorders of language, this type of aphasia comprises an isolated difficulty in evoking words as names for objects, conditions, or qualities. The problem may be so severe that speech is greatly limited. Patients with this form of aphasia are slow and hesitant in expressing themselves; in this respect they resemble individuals with expressive aphasia, but they show no difficulties in articulation. The patient with a nominal aphasia, unable to find the word for an object, hesitates and substitutes slang or colloquial expressions. Rote word series may be evoked with ease, but the patient will be unable to isolate specific items in the given series; thus, he may recite the days of the week but be unable to name the current day as a single response. An outstanding feature of this form of aphasia is the ability of the patient to recognize the word that he himself cannot produce, a characteristic not true of the expressive aphasic. Although he recognizes the correct word, and although it is repeated when proferred, the patient with nominal aphasia fails to retain the correct word. In contrast, language comprehension is good and the ability to read is preserved, although words may be omitted when he reads aloud. Writing is variably affected. Spontaneous speech is fluent. Features of a Gerstmann syndrome (see p. 123) sometimes accompany a nominal aphasia; at times defects in the visual fields appear.

The lesion responsible for a nominal aphasia is generally found in the posterior and superior portion of the dominant temporal lobe or in the vicinity of the angular gyrus.

## TRANSCORTICAL APHASIA

In contrast to the aphasias described to this point, in virtually all of which repetition is impaired, the transcortical aphasias are categorized by *intact* powers of repetition. *Transcortical motor aphasia* (anterior isolation syndrome) resembles Broca's aphasia by virtue of a predominant difficulty in expression with loss of fluency and of spontaneity, but with relatively preserved comprehension. Speech may be dysarthric, as in Broca's aphasia, and often hesitant or stuttering; a curious nonspecific somatic motor reinforcement often assists patients so afflicted to initiate speech. Reading and writing are variably affected. Of particular importance is the preservation of the ability to repeat verbal material, in contrast to the impairment of repetition characteristically seen in Broca's aphasia itself. In terms of associated abnormalities, right hemiparesis and apraxia of the left arm and leg are commonly encountered.

The lesion responsible for transcortical motor aphasia is found peripheral to the perisylvian distribution of lesions typical of the aphasic disorders described above; invariably involving the dominant frontal lobe, the lesion is ordinarily to be seen either anterior or superior to Broca's area (and, thus, in a vascular watershed distribution rather than in the prime area supplied by the middle cerebral artery itself, as is the case with all the aphasias previously discussed).

*Transcortical sensory aphasia* (posterior isolation syndrome) is characterized by the presence of marked defect in comprehension, but with striking *echolalia* (repetition of words and phrases utilized by the examiner) and with fluent although paraphrasic speech. Anomia is marked, and severe defects in both reading and writing are encountered. A hemianopic visual field defect commonly accompanies this language disorder; other neurologic disorders tend to be mild. Many patients with this form of language disorder, who exhibit such a striking ability to repeat a question but are unable to understand it, and who are without other meaningful neurologic deficits, are commonly misdiagnosed as being psychotic, particularly schizophrenic. The lesion responsible for a transcortical sensory aphasia is generally found within the posterior dominant hemisphere and involves the parieto-temporo-occipital association area; it is thus posterior to Wernicke's area itself. A *mixed* form of transcortical aphasia has also been defined and is characterized by impairment of both comprehension and expression, but with striking echolalia. Naming, reading, and writing are impaired. The lesion(s) responsible for this disorder would appear to be quite widespread and involves both anterior and posterior association areas in the vascular border zone of the dominant hemisphere.

## UNUSUAL FORMS OF APHASIA

At times a patient with a hemorrhage in the thalamus of the dominant hemisphere demonstrates a transient abnormality of language characterized by a fluent but paraphrasic speech with severe anomia, disturbance of reading and writing, preservation of comprehension, and intact repetition. This has been called a *thalamic aphasia*. Attention has also been called to a so-called *striatal aphasia* in which, following hemorrhage within the striatum of the dominant hemisphere, the patient may demonstrate a nonfluent spontaneous speech with some echolalia and marked paraphrasia but with intact comprehension of spoken language and preserved repetition. Naming and reading may be mildly impaired. The syndrome, which is generally transient, resembles particularly transcortical motor aphasia, but with unusual paraphrasic errors.

## LINGUISTIC CLASSIFICATION OF APHASIA

An alternative classification of language disorders is based on *linguistics,* that is, on the behavioral attributes of speech and identification of stages of what has been called "phonemic regression." On this basis, the several types of aphasia identified are looked upon as representing various degrees of regression, or reversal, in the normal sequence of language acquisition. Neuroanatomic criteria as such are not utilized. Although not widely accepted by clinical neurologists, this classification is sometimes utilized by others interested in problems of language, and a brief description of the more important features seems warranted here. The types of aphasia identified on the basis of this classification are as follows:

**SYNTACTIC APHASIA.** There is a loss of the grammatical function of language, with simplified, concrete, and often telegraphic speech. Little use is made of connective speech elements, and tense and gender may be improperly used. Nominal symbols, that is, substantive words, are preserved, and communication remains effective. Since the addition of syntax or grammar represents the last and highest stage in the acquisition of language, this form of aphasia represents the initial level of regression, the first stage of reversal of language function.

**SEMANTIC APHASIA.** Although grammatical form may be preserved, there is inability to relate the sign to the object (thus reminiscent of anomia). Restriction of vocabulary may be observed, and circumlocutions are prominent. Less frequently used words tend to be most severely affected. Communication is generally ineffective. This may be looked upon as dissolution of the next highest stage of language development, that of the use of substantive (naming) words.

**PRAGMATIC APHASIA.** This is a breakdown in the regulating function of language. The patient is unable to obtain meaning from stimuli and to use such stimuli as a basis for symbol formation. Speech is commonly disordered, with liberal use of paraphrasia and meaningless neologisms; the patient is unable to perceive his own errors. This seems to correspond to the stage in language development in which the child exhibits aural comprehension, but in which oral communication is for the most part fragmentary, ineffective, and contextually meaningless.

**JARGON APHASIA.** Speech here consists of a profusion of phonemically disorganized combinations of language elements, without understanding on the part of the patient. Reading and writing are impaired. This represents a reversion to the infantile stage of babbling, noncommunicative speech (prespeech).

**GLOBAL APHASIA.** This is characterized by a lack of linguistic ability, an inability to form verbal symbols for use or in comprehension. Automatic speech and echolalia are sometimes observed. In general, patients so afflicted respond little if at all to environmental stimuli and become totally dependent. Linguistically, this represents the first stage of language, that is, the infantile speechless phase, with inability to comprehend or to produce speech.

## Agnosia

Allied to the problem of aphasia are those of agnosia and apraxia. Agnosia implies the inability to recognize the form or nature of objects. It has been divided into a number of categories that are often poorly delimited one from the other. Numerous attempts have been made to localize each type to a specific portion of the cerebral hemisphere, but with varying success. Although the many forms of agnosia described in the medical literature may not in fact themselves represent clearly delineated and mutually exclusive entities, they are mentioned briefly here to acquaint the student with the more important forms encountered.

*Tactile agnosia* consists of inability to recognize objects by touch. It is commonly referred to as *astereognosis* and is typically associated with parietal lobe lesions, usually as a manifestation of a cortical sensory defect.

*Auditory agnosia* refers to inability to recognize speech sounds; the term *pure word deafness* is sometimes used for much the same disorder. Although it clearly resembles a classic Wernicke's aphasia and generally appears during recovery from such a language disorder, the responsible lesion is not necessarily the same as found with Wernicke's; bitemporal lesions or dominant subcortical temporal lesions have been described. A special form of auditory agnosia is concerned with musical sounds and is characterized by loss of the capacity to recognize tones or melodies (music deafness or *amusia*).

*Visual agnosia* has been divided into several categories, including agnosia for objects and pictures, or for human faces. The latter is referred to as *prosopagnosia* and generally reflects a lesion in the mesial temporo-occipital region, usually bilaterally; in some cases the lesion appears to be confined to the right (nondominant) hemisphere. The type of visual agnosia related specifically to written symbols is commonly called *word blindness* or verbal alexia. A dominant parietotemporal lesion appears to be important in the pathogenesis of this form of agnosia. In all varieties, there is loss of the ability to recognize objects or persons by visual cues alone; at times tactile reinforcement provides the needed additional stimulus that permits identification.

*Color agnosia* is characterized by inability to understand colors as qualities of objects, faulty color concepts, and inability to evoke color images in the absence of color blindness. It is a characteristic feature of the syndrome of alexia without agraphia (see above), which is typically encountered as a result of a lesion or lesions involving the mesial occipital lobe as well as the posterior portion of the corpus collosum.

*Spatial agnosia* may be defined as an incapacity to find one's way around familiar places, although objects in a room or house are recognized. Sometimes associated with parietal lobe lesions, this form of deficit is difficult to separate from a broader confusional state.

Other forms of agnosia are encountered in the context of disorders of the *body image* (see above). A deficit in proprioception and at least mild mental confusion seem to underlie all these syndromes. The lesions most frequently found are in the minor (nondominant) parietal lobe. *Anosognosia* consists of ignorance or denial of the existence of the disease, usually a lack of perception of a hemiplegia or other paralyzed part. The patient may believe that he can move the paralyzed part or offer a complete denial of the hemiplegia. *Autotopagnosia* (amorphosynthesis) is characterized by loss of the ability to identify the body, in whole or in part, or to recognize relationships between the various parts. The patient may, for example, feel an arm next to his body and be unaware that it is his own, or he may be unable to identify sides of the body. *Sensory inattention* may be present for tactile, visual, or auditory stimuli. In visual inattention, or extinction, the patient can see and recognize objects in any part of the visual field when called upon to do so, but will neglect that part of the visual field opposite the side of the lesion when stimuli are presented simultaneously in both halves of the visual field. A similar condition may prevail with either tactile or auditory stimuli in response to double simultaneous stimulation.

The *Gerstmann syndrome* is characterized by finger agnosia, right-left confusion, agraphia, and acalculia. Finger agnosia is expressed by difficulty in recognizing, naming, selecting, and differentiating the fingers of either hand, the patient's own as well as those of others. It involves the middle, ring, and little fingers most severely, the thumb and index less frequently and less severely, and the toes not at all. The confusion of right and left is characterized by inability to recognize sides of the body, both the patient's own and others. Acalculia appears as a difficulty, often profound, in performing even simple arithmetic problems. The full-blown syndrome is most commonly a result of a lesion involving the left (dominant) angular gyrus, in the region between the parietal and occipital cortex; when only fragments of the syndrome are recognized, however, localization of the responsible lesion is much less clear-cut.

Although not, strictly speaking, an agnosia, the syndrome of the *phantom limb* (or phantom nose, breast, penis, etc.) may be looked upon as an unawareness or lack of recognition of a loss of part of the body and, in a certain light, as an unconscious attempt to preserve the integrity of the body image. Patients so afflicted experience positive phenomena, generally tactile or proprioceptive in quality, at the site of the missing part. The limb is felt as present, though often painful and in stressful or distorted postures. With the passage of time, shrinkage and ultimately disappearance of the phantom occur. No lesions of the central nervous system are demonstrable under these circumstances; abnormal activity on the part of peripheral nerve trunks sectioned during amputation appears to be responsible for the appearance of the phantom, but the precise events leading to conscious awareness of the lost part are not known. In general, phantom limb phenomena are most prominent in instances of sudden and unanticipated loss (e.g., with traumatic amputation).

## Apraxia

This class of disorder comprises an inability to perform purposeful movements or execute the proper use of objects in the absence of significant weakness, incoordination, sensory loss, or defect in comprehension. No single anatomic substrate can be identified as a common site of lesion in patients so afflicted. Motor apraxias may be associated with a variety of aphasic disorders, which suggests that either frontal or temporal lesions are important in causation. Speech apraxia tends to be associated with an inferior frontal lesion in the dominant hemisphere, while a gait apraxia suggests bilateral hemispheral disease that involves perhaps particularly the frontal lobes. Constructional and dressing apraxias are both encountered with parietal lobe lesions, although not necessarily so; parenthetically, the use of the term apraxia for these is perhaps not entirely accurate, in that they both appear to represent basically disorders of spatial orientation and attention rather than a defect in the executive ordering of movements as such. The forms of apraxia commonly described are as follows:

*Limb kinetic apraxia* is characterized by slowness, awkwardness, and general inability to carry out a movement in the absence of paralysis.

*Ideokinetic* (ideomotor) *apraxia* is evidenced by difficulty in determining what the movement shall be, for example, inability to purse the lips, smile, raise the arm, or kick the ball to command.

*Ideational apraxia* is demonstrated by inability to recognize the specific movements necessary for the completion of a complex act and to sustain the notion of such activity. Patients so afflicted are unable to strike a match and light a cigarette, or they may strike the match on the wrong side of the box or strike with the cigarette instead of the match. More subtle defects of this type can be elicited by asking the patient to pretend to use an object, rather than actually having the object itself available.

*Constructional apraxia* causes difficulty in building with blocks, in drawing, and sometimes in writing. The patient may be aware of the faulty nature of his efforts. Design copying may similarly be affected. At times, only half the constructions or drawings are defective, almost always the left half, which indicates a primary visuospatial problem characterized by neglect of the left side of extracorporeal space.

*Dressing apraxia* is typified by failure of the patient to clothe himself correctly. As most commonly found, it is the left side that remains partially or totally unclad, as an expression of *neglect* of the left side of the body. Both dressing and constructional apraxia appear most commonly with lesions of the right, or nondominant, parietal lobe.

*Speech apraxia* has already been alluded to in the discussion of expressive (Broca's) aphasia. It is sometimes considered part of a more widespread apractic disorder called facial (orofacial, buccofacial) apraxia.

*Gait apraxia,* generally thought to be a reflection of disease of both cerebral hemispheres, particularly of the frontal lobes, consists of an inability to utilize the limbs in an effective and coordinated fashion when the patient is erect and attempting to walk. When the patient is tested in the recumbent position, however, function of the legs appears entirely normal.

*Callosal apraxia* is actually a form of ideokinetic apraxia and is characterized by normal use of the right arm and leg upon request but inability to perform the same movements with the left side when commanded to do so. A lesion in the anterior portion of the corpus collosum appears to be of significance.

## Clinical Significance of Aphasia, Agnosia, and Apraxia

Defects in language function (the aphasias) have major clinical localizing significance, since they indicate lesions in highly specific portions of the brain. As Hughlings Jackson has stated, however, "to locate the damage which destroys speech and to locate speech are two different things." Hence, the localization of lesions responsible for aphasia does not clarify the process of elaboration of speech itself. Categorically stated, expressive (Broca's) aphasia indicates a lesion in the left inferior frontal gyrus in its posterior portion and possibly also implicates the adjacent island of Reil (insula). Auditory-receptive (Wernicke's) aphasia points to a lesion in the posterior portion of the left superior temporal gyrus. Visual receptive aphasia indicates a lesion in the region of the lingual gyrus or, when found in pure form, in the splenium of the corpus collosum and the occipital cortex. In the mixed expressive-receptive (global) group, there is involvement of both frontal and temporal areas. The localization in the anomic (amnesic) group is not entirely clear, but a posterior and superior temporal locus is probable. Conduction aphasia appears to be due to a lesion in the supramarginal gyrus or one that involves the arcuate fasciculus connecting the temporal and frontal lobes. The transcortical aphasias are associated with more peripheral lesions in the frontal and parietal regions of the dominant hemisphere.

The localizing significance of the apractic and agnostic disorders is perhaps less clear-cut. In general, the lesions responsible for the agnosias are parietal or temporo-occipital. Apraxias of speech, face, and gait accompany frontal lesions particularly, whereas constructional and dressing apraxias appear as a result of parietal lobe dysfunction. Ideokinetic and ideational forms seem at times dependent on lesions of the corpus collosum for their appearance, but may be encountered with lesions of the frontal or temporal lobes as well.

The significance of isolation, or separation, of one part of the cerebrum from the remainder in the pathogenesis of disorders of this type has been re-emphasized by Geschwind, who has defined three major groups of so-called *disconnection syndromes.* The features of many of these have already been detailed; they are reiterated briefly here for the sake of clarification.

**COMMISSURAL SYNDROME.** Following destruction of all, or nearly all, of the corpus collosum surgically or as a consequence of anterior cerebral artery occlusion, a variety of clinical defects emerge, which include inability to match a stimulus object held in one hand with the other, or seen in one visual field with the other; inability to carry out verbal commands with the left hand, though able to do so with the right; inability to write with the left hand, although writing with the right hand is preserved; inability to name objects held in the left hand; inability to read in the left visual field; constructional apraxia; and abnormalities of dichotic listening. If the lesion is restricted to the splenium of the corpus collosum alone, inability to read or name objects in the left visual field may be observed as an isolated deficit.

**DISORDERS RESULTING FROM COMMISSURAL LESIONS COMBINED WITH OTHERS.**

1. Alexia without agraphia. Generally associated with a right homonymous hemianopsia and defective color naming, this syndrome appears as a result of a combination of lesions in the left visual cortex and in the splenium of the corpus collosum. So-called mind blindness, characterized by inability to identify or select objects visually, may occur with lesions similarly placed.

2. Apraxia of the left side with Broca's aphasia. A right hemiparesis is usually present as well. This defect results from a lesion that involves either the arcuate fibers as they enter the premotor region in the dominant hemisphere, or the origin of the callosal fibers. A similar clinical deficit may appear with a single large subcortical infarction.

3. Pure word deafness. This consists of difficulty in comprehension of spoken language, with normal hearing, normal identification of nonverbal sounds, and virtually normal speech, reading, and writing. It has been described under two circumstances: either as a result of bilateral lesions affecting the first temporal gyrus, or of a subcortical left temporal lobe lesion sparing Wernicke's area but implicating the left auditory radiation and the callosal fibers from the right auditory region, thus essentially disconnecting Wernicke's area from auditory stimulation.

4. Isolation of the speech area (transcortical aphasia). Comprehension and production of speech are impaired, but powers of repetition are preserved. This appears to be due to a lesion in which Wernicke's and Broca's areas, and the interconnecting arcuate fasciculus, are preserved, in the face of extensive destruction of both gray and white matter elsewhere in the dominant hemisphere.

**CONDUCTION APHASIA.** This syndrome appears particularly as a result of a lesion that interrupts intrahemispheral associational systems, specifically the internal arcuate fasciculus in the parietal operculum, the fiber system that connects Wernicke's area in the superior temporal gyrus, and Broca's area in the inferior frontal lobe; both Wernicke's and Broca's areas themselves are spared. The aphasia is fluent with paraphrasia and is associated with dysgraphia and severe impairment of the ability to repeat verbally presented phrases. Despite the disorder of repetition, the understanding of spoken and written speech is normal, or nearly so. A right hemisensory defect is found. The disorder is felt to reflect the disconnection of Wernicke's from Broca's area. Apraxia may also be observed in patients so affected, with difficulty in executing movements with either side in response to verbal commands.

## LESIONS INVOLVING THE VISUAL SYSTEM

Since a working knowledge of the anatomy of the visual conducting system is basic to an understanding of the significance of visual field abnormalities in clinical neurology, a brief review of the pathways concerned is appropriate (Fig. 3-2). It will be recalled that the visual fibers are distributed in remarkably orderly arrangement throughout their course; the great precision of this arrangement is the feature that accounts for the overwhelming importance of this system in clinical neurology. Impulses are brought to the retina from the visual field, and stimuli from the temporal field arrive at the nasal side of the retina, those from the nasal field at the temporal side. Stimuli from the upper portion of the visual field fall on the lower part of the retina and those from the lower portions on the upper part of the retina. Fibers from the temporal side of the retina (nasal

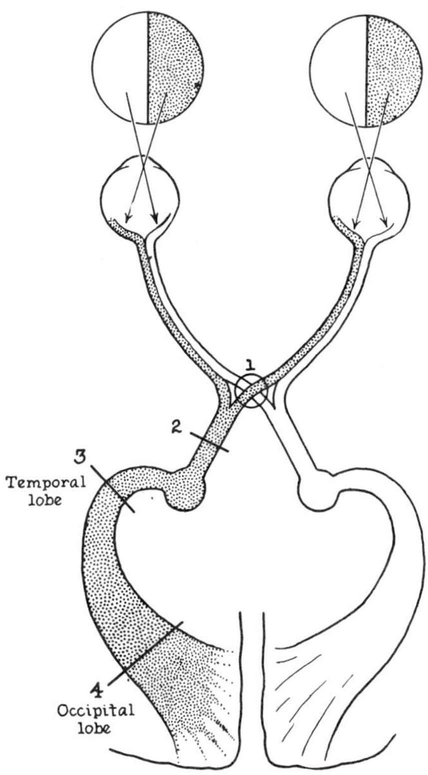


**FIGURE 3-2.** Visual fields indicating the origin and destination of the visual pathways showing the crossed and uncrossed fibers. Lesions at 1 produce bitemporal hemianopsia. Lesions at 2, 3, and 4 produce homonymous hemianopsia. Lesions at 2 and 3 are more apt to produce field cuts with involvement of the fixation points.

field) pass through the nerve and optic chiasm uncrossed, while those from the nasal side (temporal field) cross in the chiasm. In the chiasm the ratio of crossed to uncrossed fibers is 3:2. Fibers from the upper part of the retina lie in the upper part of the optic nerve and chiasm, those from the lower retina in the lower part of the optic nerve and chiasm. The visual fibers then continue to the primary optic centers, the lateral geniculate bodies. Thence they continue as the optic radiation and hook around the inferior horn of the lateral ventricle as the geniculocalcarine radiation. Here the fibers are closely packed together; they pass through the temporal and occipital lobes and fan out more and more as they proceed posteriorly to their final end stations in the upper and lower lips of the calcarine (striate) cortex of the occipital lobe. Fibers from the upper half of the retina (lower half of visual field) are distributed to the upper calcarine lip, those from the lower half of the retina (upper half of the visual field) to the lower calcarine lip.

The papillomacular bundle, which subserves central vision, runs from the macular region to the lateral geniculate body and from there to the cortex. It lies roughly in the center of the optic nerve and chiasm. Within the optic tract it tends to run superiorly and is distributed to the more superior portions of the geniculate. The macula is projected thence onto the tip of the occipital lobe; a lesion here will cause loss of central vision. Because of the frequent escape of central vision with resultant preservation of visual acuity in complete hemianopsias, it has been suggested that there is bilateral representation of the macula in the calcarine area, and it is believed by some that macular fibers cross in the splenium of the corpus collosum. Alternately, some have assumed a diffuse representation of the macula in the calcarine region. Such sparing of central vision in most hemianopsias, however, probably most frequently reflects simply a different pattern of blood supply (middle vs. posterior cerebral arteries) at the tip of the occipital lobe (macular area) as compared with the remainder of the calcarine cortex.

The form of the visual field itself is not a complete circle, since it is flattened above and restricted medially by the bony ridges of the orbit and the bridge of the nose. Its form is also affected by the width of the palpebral fissure, by the size of the pupil, and by the visual acuity. The fields are composed of binocular and monocular portions and reflect the position of the eyes in the head and the degree of overlapping of the fields of vision of each eye. Binocular portions extend out to 60° of the visual field. Beyond this, on the temporal side of each visual field, (from 60° to 90°) is a portion known as the temporal crescent, which subserves monocular vision alone.

## Visual Field Syndromes

These have already been discussed in detail (Chapter 2) and will be reviewed here only in outline form:

**SCOTOMAS.** Scotomas develop as a result of lesions of the retina, or of the optic nerve between the eye and the chiasm. They may be central, paracentral, or cecocentral. The most common is the central scotoma that is associated with retrobulbar or optic neuritis; visual acuity is decreased and color vision is impaired under these circumstances. Multiple sclerosis is a common cause, but any condition affecting the optic nerve, such as a sphenoid wing meningioma that compresses the optic nerve anterior to the chiasm, may produce a scotoma of this type.

**ALTITUDINAL ANOPIA.** This rare defect is characterized by loss of vision in the upper or lower halves of the visual field and is due to a mass lesion anterior to the optic chiasm that presses on the upper or under surfaces of the optic nerve; it may also appear in glaucoma, or with retinal detachment. Most commonly it is unilateral or monocular.

**BITEMPORAL HEMIANOPIA.** This common field defect results from compression or destruction of the decussating fibers in the center of the optic chiasm which are derived from the nasal sides of the retinae. The visual loss usually extends cleanly through the fixation point, but often with sparing of central vision. It is caused by a variety of lesions that involve the optic chiasm, chief among which are intrasellar tumors (pituitary adenomas) that have extended through the diaphragma sella, as well as primary suprasellar lesions such as meningiomas, hypophyseal stalk tumors, and aneurysms. Localized thickening of the leptomeninges, so-called chiasmatic arachnoiditis, is implicated in some cases. It is occasionally due to compression of the chiasm from above caused by a dilated third ventricle or to a third ventricle tumor. Junctional syndromes that imply simultaneous affection of an optic nerve as well as the chiasm are recognized, evidenced, for example, by a central scotoma on one side and a superior temporal defect on the other.

**BINASAL HEMIANOPIA.** A loss of both nasal fields is due to involvement of the uncrossed fibers that are derived from the temporal portions of the retinae. It results only from bilateral lesions, almost always sclerosed, tortuous, and dilated (ectatic) internal carotid arteries, but has been described with pituitary neoplasm.

**HOMONYMOUS HEMIANOPIA.** This is the most common field defect encountered. Found with lesions of all sorts that affect the optic tract and radiation, it consists of a loss of vision in the temporal field of one eye and the nasal field of the other. Homonymous hemianopia in itself has no more precise localizing value other than indicating involvement of the opposite tract or radiation, although ancillary features such as congruity or macular sparing may at times be helpful (see above). Ultimately, a clinical decision as to temporal, occipital, or parasellar (tract) involvement depends upon the presence of accompanying clinical abnormalities.

**RETINAL FIELD DEFECTS.** For purposes of comparison, brief mention may be made here of at least some of the visual defects encountered with disease of the retina itself rather than of the conducting apparatus. Conditions as divergent as neuronal storage disease (Tay-Sachs disease) or chorioretinitis may involve the macula and result in a *central scotoma* with impairment of visual acuity and of color vision. Focal destructive lesions elsewhere in the retina, as seen for example in instances of retinal hemorrhage or separation, produce delimited *sector* field cuts, which generally correspond in an anatomic sense to the diseased portion of the retina. Visual acuity is preserved as the macular area itself is spared. *Peripheral constriction* of the fields may be found in disorders that destroy retinal ganglion cells in diffuse fashion, as in methyl alcohol intoxication. A loss of night vision, or *night blindness,* is the first sign of retinitis pigmentosa, which is characterized by degeneration of the peripheral rod-bearing portions of the retina; as the disease progresses, increased limitation of the field ensues, and ultimately optic atrophy and blindness result. Night blindness is also the characteristic visual abnormality of vitamin A deficiency, and here, too, is referable to dysfunction of the rods; lack of vitamin A results in a lack of retinene and thus of rhodopsin (visual purple), the photosensitive agent of the rods.

## LESIONS OF THE UPPER MOTOR NEURON

The term upper motor neuron indicates any central neuron conveying impulses to the anterior horn cell(s). Lesions may affect this nerve cell anywhere in its course from the cerebrum to the anterior horn cell of the spinal cord. The most important pathway concerned is the corticospinal (pyramidal) tract (Fig. 3-3), which takes its origin in the motor cells of the frontal cortex, passes through the internal capsule, cerebral peduncle, and pons, decussates almost completely low in the medulla, passes down the cord in the lateral column, and forms a synapse eventually with anterior horn cells. The uncrossed portion of the corticospinal tract, accounting for perhaps 15 percent of the corticospinal fibers, descends in the anterior compartment of the cord. Not all the fibers of the corticospinal or pyramidal tract are derived from the Betz cells of the precentral gyrus; however, the exact contribution from other portions of the cerebrum remains in dispute. Fibers originating in the precentral gyrus, and in the parietal lobe, account for 50 percent of the axons in the pyramid. Whether the remaining 50 percent of fibers are of cortical or subcortical origin is uncertain; since about half the fibers in the pyramid remain intact after hemispherectomy, it is clear that subcortical levels contribute a major portion thereof. In this connection, it is interesting additionally to note that there are only 25,000 to 30,000 Betz cells in the motor cortex, whereas there are approximately 1 million axons in the pyramid. Only about 10 to 15 percent of the fibers in the pyramidal tract actually achieve direct synaptic connection with anterior horn cells; the majority end in relation to cells in the intermediate zone. On the other hand, a variety of

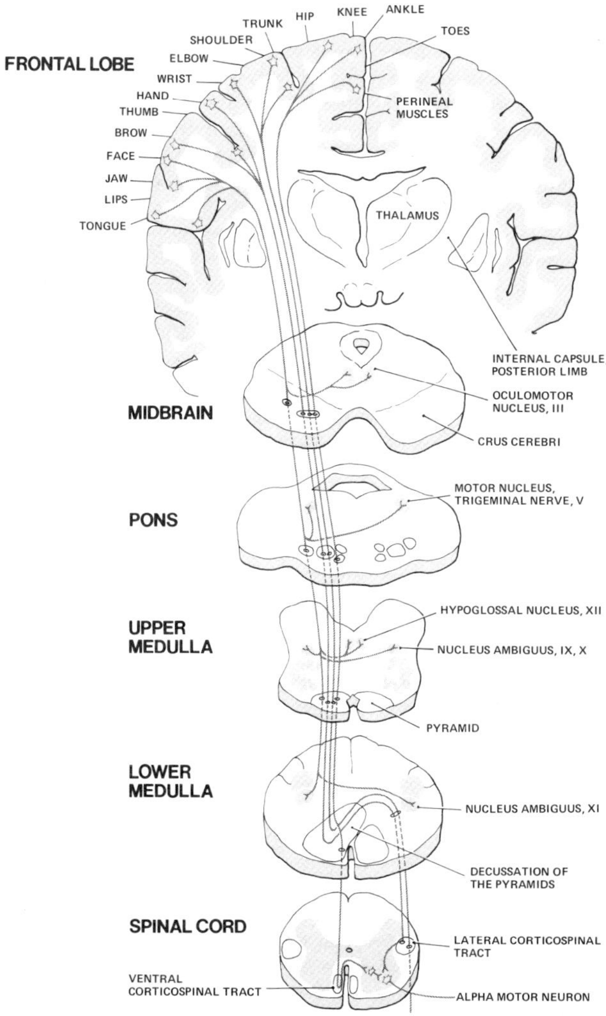


**FIGURE 3-3.** Corticospinal tract indicating its origin and destination around the anterior horn cells.

other nonpyramidal upper motor neuron impulses play upon the anterior horn cell, carried in the rubrospinal, tectospinal, reticulospinal, and olivospinal pathways.

Interruption of the corticospinal pathway results in paralysis of the opposite side of the body; this is known as hemiplegia (complete paralysis) or hemiparesis (weakness). The face may or may not participate, depending upon the segmental level of the lesion responsible. When both corticospinal pathways are interrupted in the brain, *diplegia* results, as in the cerebral diplegia of childhood. With a lesion below the brainstem, one may observe either *paraplegia,* involving usually the legs, or *quadriplegia,* when all four limbs are affected.

The term paraplegia is customarily used to refer to paralysis or weakness of the legs, but it can be used for paralysis of the arms as well (brachial paraplegia). It is associated as a rule with bilateral pyramidal tract disease in the spinal cord below the level of the cervical enlargement. It may on occasion result from focal bilateral disease of the cerebrum itself, as in instances of parasagittal meningioma, or even of the corticospinal pathways in the brainstem. In the majority of cases of paraplegia, the legs are maintained in a posture of extension. In some instances of both spinal and cerebral disease, however, and perhaps as a manifestation of persistent extrapyramidal activity, a *paraplegia in flexion* develops. In such cases, the legs exhibit involuntary flexor spasms, which are elicited by such nonspecific stimulation as touching the foot or stroking the skin. Initially, these flexor spasms are followed by involuntary extension, which results in an irregular pattern of alternating flexion and extension posturing. Eventually, such a pattern gives way to a complete, fixed flexion paraplegia. In the final stages of the disorder, the legs are paralyzed; the patellar reflexes cannot be elicited because of the marked flexor rigidity and contractures; and the withdrawal reflexes are greatly exaggerated.

When paraplegia develops acutely, as in cases of spinal cord injury or in acute transection from other causes, flaccidity is the rule, as a manifestation of the syndrome of *spinal shock.* Spasticity ordinarily ensues with the passage of time. A spastic paraplegia is ordinarily easily recognized when the patient walks because the gait is characteristically stiff and shuffling as a result of the increased extensor tonus. On recumbency, spasticity usually persists, but may disappear to appear once again when the patient walks. If only a portion of the corticospinal pathway is affected, *monoplegia* may result. This is manifested by loss of power in a restricted distribution on the opposite side of the body. Isolated facial weakness may appear, or weakness of a hand (manual monoplegia), of an arm (brachial monoplegia), or of face, tongue, and arm, (facial-lingual-brachial monoplegia). The number of possible combinations is great and depends upon the exact area affected. Monoplegias almost always result from disease of the motor cortex, but in rare instances they reflect involvement of the descending corticospinal pathway.

## Signs of Upper Motor Lesions

Upper motor lesions are characterized by the following constellation of symptoms.

### PARALYSIS

In a typical instance this involves the opposite arm, leg and side of the face; the precise distribution reflects the site of the lesion. In some cases the palate and tongue are affected, and in an acute hemiplegia, the chest and abdominal muscles on the affected side are implicated. The paralysis is usually *spastic* and, thus, in sharp contrast to the flaccid paralysis of lower motor neuron disease. It is characterized by an increase of muscle tone of a "clasp-knife" variety: attempted passive movement results first in an increase of tone, followed, as one continues, by a sudden relief. In some cases, a uniform resistance is present throughout the range of passive movement. With the ordinary spastic hemiparesis, the affected limbs assume a characteristic attitude, with varying degrees of flexion of the elbow, wrist, and fingers, pronation of the forearm, and adduction of

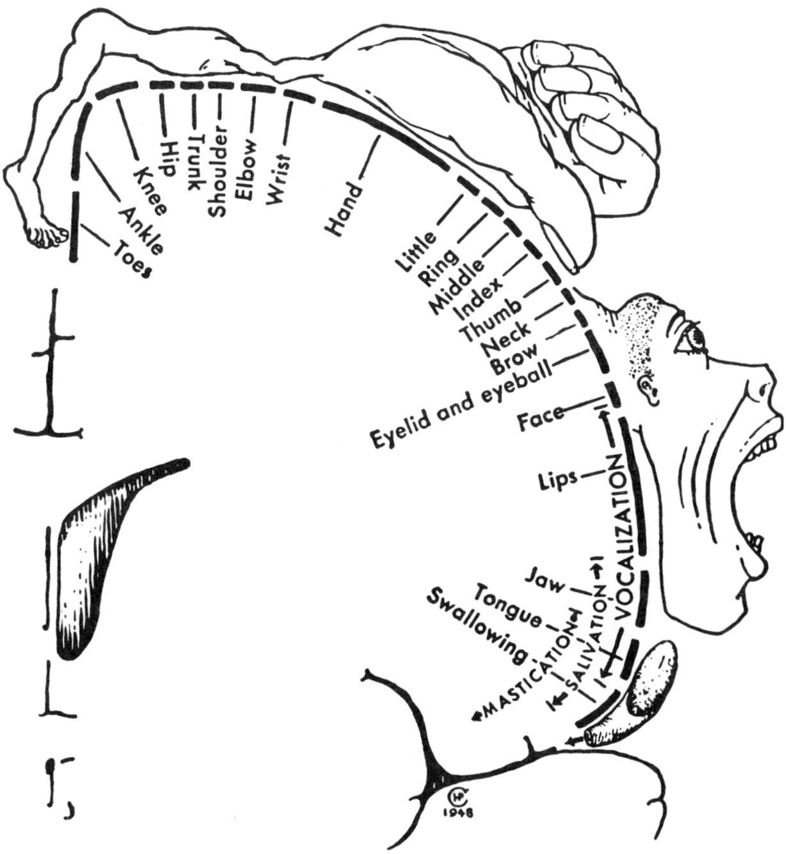


**FIGURE 3-4.** Motor homunculus, showing the representation of the various parts of the body in the motor cortex. The face, hand, and foot areas are most widely represented. (From Penfield, W., and Rasmussen, T.: *The Cerebral Cortex of Man: A Clinical Study of Localization of Function.* 1950. By permission of the Macmillan Co.)

the shoulder, along with an extended posture of the leg. Typically, the distal muscles are involved by weakness to a greater extent than the proximal; thus, in the arm, finger and hand movements are severely affected and movements of the forearm, upper arm, and shoulder much less so. With discrete lesions in the motor cortex, however, very focal deficits may appear, which reflect the precise somatotopic representation evident here (Fig. 3-4); one may encounter, for example, a proximal pattern of weakness with so-called watershed infarction. Topographical representation is also found in the internal capsule (Fig. 3-5), and small lesions here may result in restricted clinical deficits.

Paralysis caused by interruption of the corticospinal tract is not always spastic; as has been pointed out, it may be flaccid in the face of an acutely evolving lesion. Under such circumstances, the flaccidity may be transient or permanent. The cause of flaccidity with upper motor neuron lesions is not definitely known, and its occurrence with lesions of the cerebral hemispheres constitutes a thorny problem. Experimentally, lesions restricted to the motor strip itself result in flaccid paralysis. Spasticity appears only when the lesion extends anteriorly to involve much of the premotor frontal cortex, a portion of the cortex with well-established projections to a variety of deep "extrapyramidal" nuclear aggregates, for example, striatum, substantia nigra, subthalamic nucleus, red nucleus, reticular formation, and pontine nuclei. Strictly comparable data are not available for man, since pure motor or premotor cortical lesions are very rare. Spastic hemiplegia is more commonly encountered in humans and appears most frequently associated with deep lesions involving the centrum semiovale or internal capsule. The available evidence would thus suggest that spasticity resulting from lesions of the corticospinal system is actually due to unopposed, or released, activity of some other, extra-

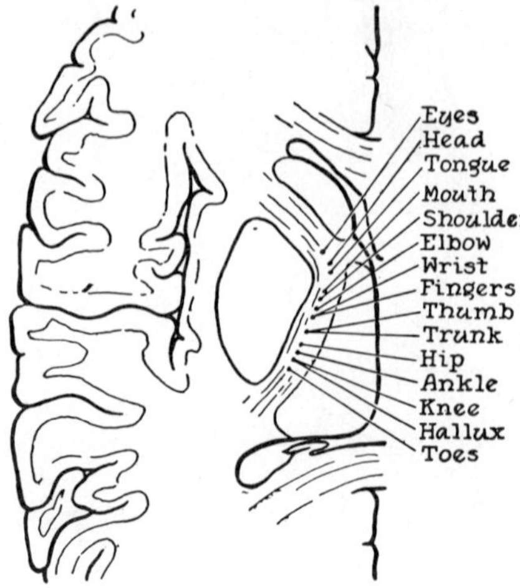


**FIGURE 3-5.** Internal capsule, showing in diagram form the situation of the fibers to the various portions of the limbs and trunk of the opposite side of the body.

pyramidal, part of the brain and therefore a manifestation of extrapyramidal rather than pyramidal activity. Walshe's comment remains appropriate: "From clinical and experimental sources come several indications, as yet imperfectly understood, that a pure cortical lesion of the pyramidal system often does not produce spasticity as an accompaniment of the loss of power. They suggest the possibility that in the cerebral lesion underlying, for example, a typical spastic residual hemiplegia, analysis may ultimately reveal a second component. That is, in addition to a negative lesion of the corticospinal path, interruption of another descending path may be concerned in the production of spasticity. Such a path need not necessarily be cerebrospinal."

## BULBAR AFFECTION AND HEMIPLEGIA

With corticospinal lesions above the level of mid-pons, facial paralysis appears as a so-called "central" facial weakness. It involves the lower part of the face and is evidenced by slowness and weakness in retraction of the mouth and flattening of the normal angulation of the mouth and of the nasolabial fold on the affected side. The palate may also be paralyzed, which is manifested by drooping of the affected side and pulling of the palate up to the healthy side on phonation. The tongue may be similarly

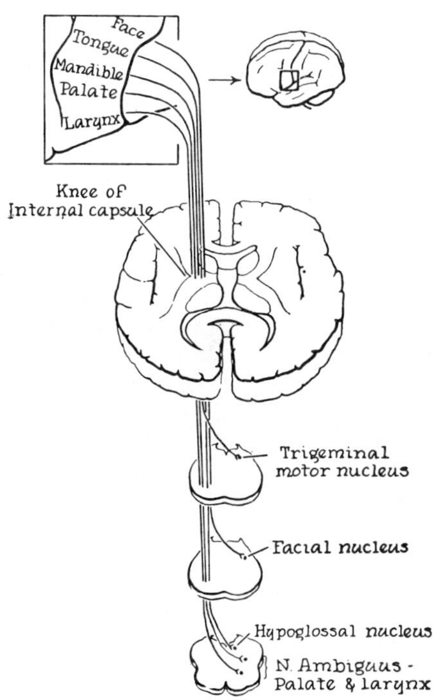


**FIGURE 3-6.** Corticobulbar tract, showing the projection of the corticobulbar pathways on the motor nuclei of the brainstem.

involved, with deviation to the paralyzed side on protrusion. The mechanism of production of cranial nerve palsies in hemiplegia is understandable by reference to pertinent anatomic relationships. The motor nuclei of the brainstem receive innervation from the motor cortex through the corticobulbar tract, which runs with, but is distinct from, the corticospinal system (Fig. 3-6). Fibers to the face are conveyed through this tract, with the forehead and eyelids being innervated bilaterally, while the lower portion of the face receives only unilateral innervation; for this reason only the lower portion of the face is paralyzed as a result of a unilateral corticospinal lesion. Most other bulbar motor functions, such as phonation and chewing, receive bilateral innervation and are, therefore, spared in unilateral corticospinal/corticobulbar disease; movement of the palate and tongue, however, may be affected.

## INCREASE OF STRETCH REFLEXES

The muscle stretch reflexes of the paralyzed side (biceps, triceps, patellar, Achilles) are overactive in corticospinal lesions, presumably as the result of release of the anterior horn cells from the inhibitory effects, direct or indirect, of the corticospinal pathway. Generally speaking, the reflexes are increased in proportion to the spasticity, but not invariably so. Muscles may be so spastic as to prevent an adequate reflex response; on the other hand, a flaccid hemiplegia may be associated with overactive reflexes.

## CLONUS

Clonus is frequently found along with increased muscle tone and hyperreflexia in corticospinal tract disease. It consists of repetitive movement of the muscles, a rhythmic reappearance of contraction after stimulation. Ankle clonus is most commonly seen, but patellar, wrist, finger, and even pectoral clonus may be encountered. Ankle clonus is elicted by quick, vigorous dorsiflexion of the foot with the knee held in flexion. The result sought for in cases of corticospinal disease is a repeated ("clonic") movement of the foot maintained so long as the foot is held firmly in dorsiflexion. Ordinarily, the clonus stops when the foot is released, but it may continue spontaneously and cease only with vigorous plantar flexion. Spontaneous clonus at the ankle may develop in cases of advanced spasticity. Patellar clonus is elicited by vigorous downward movement of the patella, with the leg in full extension; wrist clonus, by vigorous extension of the wrist.

## LOSS OF CUTANEOUS REFLEXES

A common but certainly not invariable feature of corticospinal disease is the loss of the cutaneous reflexes, notably the abdominal and cremasteric, on the side of the paralysis. They are lost bilaterally in paraplegia. The corneal reflex may also be decreased or lost in acute hemiplegia and return with recovery. The mechanism of loss of the superficial reflexes under these circumstances is not well understood. The basic reflex arc concerned at least in loss of the abdominal, and presumably the cremasteric, reflex would appear to be spinal. Since there is no evidence of abnormality at the spinal or peripheral level in the typical hemiplegia, it must be assumed that the decrease in response is due to an alteration in balance of excitatory and inhibitory influences at segmental levels by withdrawal of innervation from above.

## PATHOLOGIC REFLEXES

The most important of the abnormal reflexes found in patients with corticospinal disease is the extensor plantar response of Babinski (Babinski's sign). This is pathognomonic of corticospinal disease. Although Babinski's sign never occurs without corticospinal disease, at least after infancy, the converse is not necessarily true and the typical response may in fact be lacking in well-established disorder of the corticospinal tract. This and other pathologic responses have been described in detail in Chapter 2.

In many cases, all signs are easily elicited. As indicated, however, they may be present in various combinations. Subtle alterations in these parameters may be quite important. Thus, only slight weakness of one side may be present (hemiparesis), and associated with only minimally increased reflexes, with or without abnormal reflexes; or there may be a Babinski sign without other evidence of corticospinal disease; or weakness may be present with normal reflexes. Of all of these, it is the positive Babinski (extensor plantar) response that invariably means corticospinal disease, even as an isolated observation.

It is often necessary to differentiate a hemiplegia of structural (i.e., organic) origin from one of psychogenic causation. Of basic importance of course is the personality structure, which is often found to be consistent with a psychogenic reaction. The history is often helpful, particularly in regard to onset of the weakness and the circumstances surrounding it. Most important, however, are the discrepancies revealed on examination. There may be good finger dexterity despite hand weakness; balancing on the weak leg may be quite normal; walking may fail to reveal the typical hemiplegic or hemiparetic gait; the weak arm may have no difficulty in performing rapid alternating or patting tests; the reflexes may not be increased; and there may be no pathologic reflexes.

# LESIONS OF THE LOWER MOTOR NEURON

Lesions of the lower motor neuron may involve the anterior horn cells, the anterior roots, or the peripheral nerve, that is, the peripheral neuron anywhere in its course from its cell body of origin (anterior horn cell) outward. Common symptoms of deficit arise whether the interruption involves the anterior horn cell itself, the root, or the motor nerve. It may prove possible to differentiate the various levels of involvement on clinical grounds, but it must be stressed that the majority of the clinical features are identical regardless of the site of affection. All such lesions produce paralysis, atrophy, reflex loss, and changes in the electromyogram. There are, however, certain distinguishing features that permit clinical distinctions to be drawn in terms of specific syndromes of lower motor neuron dysfunction.

## Anterior Horn Cell Syndrome

The features of anterior horn cell disease, or of disease of the motor cranial nerve nuclei, are the same regardless of the specific disease process concerned (poliomyelitis, amyotrophic lateral sclerosis, progressive muscular atrophy, syringomyelia, etc.). The syndrome is characterized by a number of features. *Paralysis* is always flaccid and segmental in character and its extent is determined by the number of anterior horn cells destroyed. *Atrophy* is always present and its severity reflects the degree of loss of nerve cells. It may appear soon after the paralysis occurs or may be delayed. *Loss of reflexes* follows from interruption of the efferent limb of the reflex arc. *Fasciculations* occur typically as part of the anterior horn cell syndrome, but may occasionally be observed when the lesion involves more peripheral portions of the lower motor neuron. Even in the face of anterior horn cell disease, fasciculations may be lacking by virtue of total atrophy of the muscle, or they may be obscured by overlying fat. *Absence of sensory disturbances* is noted, since the anterior horn cells are entirely motor in function. *Fibrillation potentials and other evidence of denervation* are demonstrated by electromyographic testing.

The pathogenesis of the various features of disease of the anterior horn cells is a matter of practical interest. The *paralysis* is the direct result of loss of innervation of the muscles caused by interruption of the motor fibers at their cell of origin. It is obvious that if all the cells innervating a muscle or muscles are destroyed, the paralysis will be complete; if the anterior horn cell destruction is incomplete, the degree of paralysis will depend upon the number of cells destroyed and, therefore, the number of fibers interrupted. Study of the innervation ratio, that is, the proportion of nerve to muscle fibers in lower animals, indicates that in extensor longus digitorum, for example, the ratio is 1:165, and in soleus 1:120. This means that when one anterior horn cell to the soleus is stimulated, an average of 120 muscle fibers is activated; consequently the loss of even a single anterior horn cell may result in appreciable loss of power in the affected muscle. A single anterior horn cell can also be shown capable, with repetitive discharge, of developing an average of 30 g of tension in the gastrocnemius, another indication of the significance of a single cell in this regard.

An important characteristic of paralysis caused by anterior horn cell disease is its *segmental character.* The spinal cord is a chain of segments operating through separate reflex arcs interacting with one another, each segment bearing a well-defined relationship to a specific sensory and motor segment of the body. On the motor side, specific muscles are innervated through a single cord segment or, as is more usual, through two or three segments. Thus, segments C5 and C6 in the cervical cord innervate the biceps, deltoid, part of the pectoralis major, teres major and minor, serratus magnus, supraspinatus, infraspinatus, rhomboids, subscapularis, and the flexor muscles of the hand. A lesion involving these segments, therefore, will result in complete or partial paralysis of the affected muscles or, in essence, a segmental type of paralysis. The same group of muscles may of course be affected by simultaneous involvement of their respective peripheral nerves, but the resulting features differ substantially from those of anterior horn cell disease. It does not, however, necessarily follow that in disease of a specific segment or segments all the muscles innervated through these segments will be paralyzed, or that all muscles affected will be so to an equal degree. Considerable variability in these parameters is observed in clinical practice.

The *atrophy* resulting from anterior horn cell disease remains unexplained in many respects. Intact innervation is clearly essential for the maintenance of normal muscle bulk, and, thus, anatomic continuity of the nerve is important in preventing atrophy. It has been suggested that atrophy results from the overactivity of the muscle as a result of constant fasciculations or fibrillations following denervation; however, drugs that reduce such activity (quinidine, atropine) or increase it (acetylcholine, neostigmine) equally fail to evidence a recognizable effect. Electrical stimulation is recognizably effective in delaying atrophy; it follows that maintenance of muscle tension and activity is of great importance in preventing atrophy. The time of development of atrophy after anterior horn cell disease varies considerably; it may develop rapidly, as in poliomyelitis, or more slowly, as in progressive muscular atrophy or amyotrophic lateral sclerosis. From a clinical standpoint, the extent of atrophy seems to parallel the destruction of anterior horn cells; atrophy may, however, be so diffuse as to obscure its segmental nature.

## Anterior Root Syndrome

This syndrome is virtually indistinguishable from that of the anterior horns, although fasciculations tend to be less prominent. When the posterior roots are involved simultaneously, as is often the case in human extramedullary disease, radicular pain becomes an important accompaniment.

## Motor Peripheral Nerve Syndrome

Some peripheral nerves are exclusively or almost exclusively motor in function (e.g., radial, long thoracic nerve). Disease of such nerves gives rise to manifestations basically similar to those of anterior horn cell disease. The main clinical characteristics are (1) paralysis, flaccid in all peripheral nerve syndromes; (2) atrophy of the muscle or muscles supplied by the affected nerve; (3) loss of reflexes; (4) absence of sensory disturbance; (5) absence of pain; and (6) electromyographic evidence of denervation. They differ, however, in some respects. Thus, the atrophy with peripheral nerve disease is as a rule less extensive and severe and develops less rapidly. With complete transection of the nerve, however, atrophy may be fully as intense as observed in anterior horn cell disease. Additionally fasciculations are ordinarily not seen in disease of the peripheral nerves; when encountered, the assumption is often made that there is coexistent anterior horn cell disease.

## Mixed Peripheral Nerve Syndrome

Since most nerves contain both motor and sensory fibers, disorders involving the peripheral nerves are most commonly of a mixed type. Not all the features of a mixed peripheral nerve syndrome are found to the same degree in all instances of involvement of the nerve, or nerves; variability depends upon such factors as the nature of the causative agent and the degree of damage to the nerve. A number of clinical features are characteristically encountered in a disease of mixed peripheral nerves:

1. Pain. When present this immediately differentiates the syndrome from pure anterior horn cell or motor root affection. Pain may be quite intense, as in alcoholic (nutritional) or diabetic neuropathy, or with peripheral nerve tumors; many neuropathies, however, are relatively painfree. When present, pain is experienced in the distribution of the peripheral nerve affected. It is usually constant and quite severe. At times, especially when there has been only partial disruption of a peripheral nerve, an intractable, virtually constant complex of pain and dysesthesiae appears, known as *causalgia*. This is frequently accompanied by evidence of autonomic dysfunction in the distribution of the damaged nerve.

2. Tenderness of the nerves and muscles. Tenderness of the nerves is almost always present, but varies in degree and intensity. Muscle tenderness is usually present in the region of the muscles supplied by the affected nerve. While nerve and muscle tenderness is always found in conditions of irritation of a mixed nerve, it may also be noted as a result of compression of a nerve or nerve root at a distance, as in herniated lumbar disc and spinal cord tumor.

3. Paralysis. This is flaccid in nature and depends in degree on the amount of injury to the nerve or nerves concerned.

4. Atrophy. Loss of muscle bulk is usually present, but varies in de-

gree; the principles governing the degree of atrophy in anterior horn cell disease hold true for peripheral nerves as well.

5. Loss or diminution of reflexes.
6. Electromyographic evidence of denervation.
7. Sensory disturbances. These appear in the appropriate peripheral nerve distribution involving all types of sensation, both deep and superficial, in complete interruption, and only superficial sensation (pain, touch, heat, cold) in other cases, and generally in unpredictable combinations. Hyperesthesiae, dysesthesiae, or paresthesiae may all be experienced in disease of mixed peripheral nerves as well.

## LESIONS OF THE EXTRAPYRAMIDAL SYSTEM

The extrapyramidal system is that portion of the motor apparatus composed of the basal ganglia and those parts of the cerebral cortex that possess motor functions but are not part of the corticospinal (pyramidal) system. There is controversy over precisely which subcortical nuclear masses should be included, but the following are generally agreed upon: caudate, putamen, globus pallidus, subthalamic nucleus (Luysii), red nucleus, substantia nigra. Some include the thalamus and hypothalamus, as well as the cerebellum and the deep cerebellar, pontine, and olivary nuclei. All nuclei so included are richly connected with one another, but their precise functional inter-relationships are not fully understood. From the clinical point of view, disease of the extrapyramidal system in the broadest sense results in disturbance of movement, as would be surmised from the motor function of the system as a whole. Such disturbances are of three sorts: akinetic or hypokinetic; hyperkinetic; mixed. Weakness *per se* is not a feature of extrapyramidal disease, and other characteristics of motor neuron disease (e.g., atrophy, reflex alteration, fasciculations) are generally lacking.

### Akinetic or Hypokinetic Syndrome

The term akinesia, or hypokinesia, refers to a poverty of movements, which sometimes amounts to complete immobility. Slowness of volitional movement *(bradykinesia)* is observed as well as difficulty in initiating movements on request. Heightened muscle tone, in particular rigidity, is characteristically encountered. Paralysis agitans (Parkinson's disease) epitomizes this type of disorder and may be used for illustrative purposes. Briefly, the parkinsonian patient exhibits muscular rigidity of cogwheeling type. When the forearm is slowly pronated and supinated, or flexed and extended, the movement is felt by the observer as a series of catches and releases, as if a muscle were being moved over a cog (hence the term "cogwheel sign"). Resistance tends to be uniform throughout the range of passive motion. There is marked poverty of movement of the face (and, thus, the masked facies and infrequent blinking typical of the disease), and of the limbs. In advanced cases, virtual immobility is the rule. The movements that are carried out are generally slow, and few accessory movements are discerned. The head and trunk are held in a flexed posture, the face is fixed, the speech is low and monotonous, and the gait is slow and shuffling with small steps *(marche à petits pas)* and without the normal associated swinging movements of the arms. It is tempting to relate such hypokinetic or akinetic phenomena to the muscular rigidity itself, but this is not necessarily the case, since the degree of akinesia and the severity of the rigidity need not parallel each other. A hyperkinetic element in the form of a resting tremor is often present as well. Along with the reduced motility, slowing of mentation (bradyphrenia) is common in parkinsonian patients. On occasion a severe dementia appears; with specific and detailed testing, at least mild intellectual impairment is the rule. The reflexes are usually normal, and no Babinski sign is found.

## Hyperkinetic Syndromes

### CHOREIFORM SYNDROME

This is seen most characteristically in the acute chorea of Sydenham and in the chronic progressive chorea of Huntington. It is evidenced by rapid, discrete, random, and purposeless involuntary movements affecting the face, limbs, and trunk, and occasionally the diaphragm. Facial grimacing is common. Chorea is observed typically in degenerative disease of the striatum, as in Huntington's disease; the pathologic substrate of Sydenham's (rheumatic) chorea or chorea gravidarum, or of the drug-related (i.e., toxic) choreas caused, for example, by agents as diverse as levodopa or phenytoin, is not clearly established. Choreiform movements have also been recorded on occasion with disease of many portions of the brain, including cortex, thalamus, red nucleus, and subthalamic nucleus; care must be taken, however, to exclude myoclonic jerks (as with diffuse cortical disease) or ballistic movements (as with focal lesions of the subthalamic nucleus) from consideration. Chorea may be unilateral *(hemichorea)* and sufficiently violent at times to be confused with hemiballismus caused by unilateral disease of the subthalamic nucleus. With recovery from a hemiplegia, choreic movements, called *posthemiplegic chorea,* may develop in the affected limbs, as well as in the face; the occurrence of this syndrome has not been explained satisfactorily, although it is often attributed to residual sensory deficits.

The facial grimacing of chorea may be difficult or impossible to distinguish from the orofacial movements of *tardive dyskinesia,* a movement disorder that appears especially following the protracted use of phenothiazines. This movement disorder, which develops with particular frequency in the elderly and in females, appears to be due to induced postsynaptic dopamine hypersensitivity. Even with discontinuation of the responsible neuroleptic, and despite vigorous therapy with a wide range of drugs, the movements once induced may persist indefinitely. In the elderly, movements identical to those of drug-induced tardive dyskinesia may appear without antecedent drug usage in the syndrome of *senile chorea.*

## ATHETOID SYNDROME

Athetoid movements are, in contrast to chorea, irregular, slow and sinuous movements, most evident in the distal portion of the limbs, especially in the digits. Facial grimacing and movements of the head commonly accompany the movements of the limbs. Writhing movements of the tongue are frequent; speech and swallowing may be disturbed by virtue of involvement of the pharyngeal muscles. The responsible lesion in cases of athetosis appears to lie in the basal ganglia, although the exact areas involved are not definitely established. Ablation of the motor and premotor cortex results in permanent extinction of athetosis in some cases, in temporary extinction in others; both chorea and athetosis tend to disappear after the spontaneous development of hemiplegia. Athetosis appears in many circumstances, both congenital and acquired, including, for example, the so-called double athetosis of childhood, Huntington's disease, Wilson's disease, and carbon monoxide encephalopathy. It is often combined with chorea, as so-called choreoathetosis.

*Pseudoathetosis* is encountered with disease of the posterior columns or dorsal roots and reflects loss of proprioception. It consists primarily of groping extensor movements of the fingers. Pseudoathetosis may appear in a variety of disorders, including tabes, subacute combined degeneration of the cord, and multiple sclerosis, or, indeed, with any disease of the central or peripheral nervous system in which position sense is lost.

## DYSTONIC SYNDROME

Even slower than athetoid movements are those of dystonia, which are slow, agonizing, writhing, virtually serpentine movements that generally involve the proximal musculature of the limbs and of the neck and trunk. Such spasms sometimes seem to spread from the distal portion of the limbs to the proximal. Facial grimacing often accompanies the dystonic movements of the limbs. The term dystonia is also applied to the abnormal *posture* of the limbs commonly found in disorders of the basal ganglia. The precise location of the lesions in the basal ganglia responsible for the appearance of dystonic movements is not clear; the caudate and putamen are most commonly implicated. This hyperkinetic disorder is seen in most striking form in that familial disorder called *dystonia musculorum deformans,* or torsion spasm, a disorder that appears in childhood, with a strong genetic basis, and occurs typically though not invariably among Ashkenazic Jews. A less severe form of the disorder involves adults, is sporadic in development, and tends to be less severe.

Dystonia may also appear in a variety of other circumstances, for example, after carbon monoxide poisoning, in Parkinson's disease, as a residual of kernicterus, or acutely as a manifestation of an idiosyncratic reaction to phenothiazines, among other neuroleptics. Dystonic movements involving especially the face, head, and neck may appear as a complication of levodopa therapy, and dystonia may also appear as an untoward side effect of the use of phenytoin. *Spasmodic torticollis* is sometimes looked upon as a fragmentary dystonic syndrome, as is the syndrome of *writer's cramps* and other focal disorders of this type, including so-called *laryngopharyngeal dystonia* and the syndrome of *blepharospasm-oromandibular dystonia* (Brueghel's syndrome).

## DISTURBANCES OF COORDINATION

Three neural systems participate in the production of smooth, coordinated movements: the posterior columns, the cerebellum, and the vestibular system. All are part of the proprioceptive system and all have important functions in the maintenance of posture: the vestibular system acts through the labyrinthine and righting reflexes; the posterior columns, through the proprioceptors of muscles, tendons, and joints; and the cerebellum, through its action in synergizing movements. Impulses transmitted through the posterior column system reach consciousness, while those mediated via the cerebellar pathways do not do so directly. The former may be regarded, therefore, as the conscious element of the proprioceptive system, and the latter, as its unconscious portion. Dysfunction in any of these systems results in disturbance of coordination, movement, and equilibrium.

### Syndrome of the Posterior Column System

The posterior columns (fasciculi of gracilis and cuneatus) run the length of the spinal cord; the gracilis (or column of Goll) extends from the midthoracic cord inferiorly and conveys impulses from the legs and lower trunk, and the cuneatus (or column of Burdach) extends from the midthoracic region superiorly and conveys impulses from the arms and upper trunk. The fibers from these columns synapse in the medulla; following decussation, the second order fibers rise thence as the mesial fillet (or lemniscus) to the thalamus, from which, after synapsing once again, they proceed on to the cerebral (parietal) cortex. They convey deep sensations from the muscles, joints, and tendons, which are measured clinically chiefly by proprioception sense and vibration sense. Impulses conveyed through the system thus provide information regarding position of the limbs in space and the force and range of movement. Additionally, this system comprises one of the pathways concerned with touch sensation and two-point discrimination.

In disease involving the posterior columns the degree of deficit and, thus, of the resulting symptoms depends on the severity and extent of the damage pathologically. The clinical manifestations typically have the following characteristics: (1) They are dependent on sensory deficit, notably impairment or loss of muscle and position sense. By and large, the more severe the deficit, the more severe the symptoms. (2) They are basically the same regardless of where the lesion is located along the pathway from cord to cortex, although some differences appear with cortical lesions. (3) Increase in symptoms follows elimination of vision.

*Ataxia* is the outstanding symptom of lesions involving the posterior column system. It is dependent on loss of position sense and is typically increased by eliminating visual impulses. Thus, the ataxia of posterior column disease is increased with the eyes closed as in the Romberg test, and in the dark, as observed in the gait disturbance in diseases such as tabes or subacute combined degeneration of the cord. Patients with posterior column disease must watch the movements of the legs in walking, and of the arms in reaching. A characteristic feature of this form of ataxia is the appearance of errors in range of movement, or *dysmetria.* Smooth, coordinated movements become impossible, and movements such as placing the finger on the nose, or the heel on the knee, overshoot the mark, usually with gross irregularity of movement. Dysmetria seen under these circumstances reflects an inability to gauge the position of limbs in space and is thus dependent on sensory (proprioceptive) deficit. The severity of the ataxia and of the dysmetria is usually in direct proportion to the loss of position sense. It should, of course, be pointed out that loss of vibratory sense alone, without concomitant loss of position sense, does not result in ataxia.

The ataxic symptoms that result from defective proprioception are the most striking features of posterior column disease. However, other manifestations are also noted, including particularly astereognosis and disturbance of two-point discrimination.

Posterior column dysfunction occurs in a wide variety of conditions and exhibits the same clinical characteristics no matter what the underlying pathologic state. It is found in subacute combined degeneration of the cord, multiple sclerosis, cord tumor, and with a host of other intrinsic diseases of the spinal cord; similar features also appear in disease of the posterior roots, such as tabes dorsalis. As already indicated, the symptoms of posterior column affection are the same regardless of the point of interruption of the system, whether in cervical or lumbar cord, in the mesial lemniscus in the brainstem, or in the thalamus.

## Syndrome of the Cerebellar System

The cerebellum (Fig. 3-7) is intimately concerned with coordination of movement and maintenance of posture. It has wide connections with virtually all parts of the neuraxis. Thus, it receives impulses from the trunk and limbs through the spinocerebellar pathways and from the head and

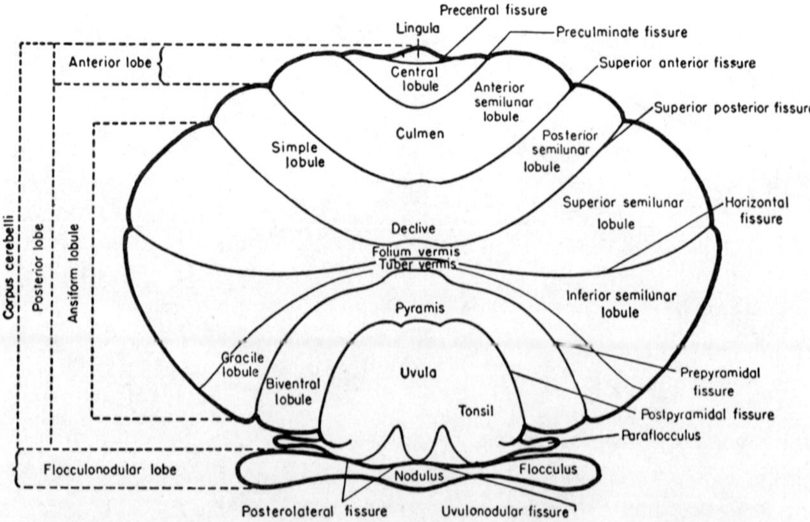


**FIGURE 3-7.** A diagram of the human cerebellum. (From Larsell, O.: *Anatomy of the Nervous System.* ed. 2. 1951. Courtesy of Appleton-Century-Crofts, Inc. Reproduced from Peele, T. L.: *The Neuroanatomical Basis for Clinical Neurology..*

neck via the external cuneate fibers. It has an intimate association with the vestibular system, basal ganglia, and the tectum, and has important though indirect connections with the cerebral cortex via the pontine nuclei. A number of nuclear aggregates of the brainstem, such as the olivary, arcuate, and reticular nuclei, also exhibit significant anatomic relationships. The vast majority of the afferent fibers enter the cerebellum through the inferior and middle cerebellar peduncles (restiform body and brachium pontis). The principle efferent pathway is the superior cerebellar peduncle (brachium conjunctivum), which carries dentato-rubro-thalamic fibers that effect widespread connections in the brainstem, basal ganglia, and thalamus.

The precise pathophysiologic mechanism underlying the development of clinical manifestations in patients with cerebellar disease remains a matter of dispute. Defective maintenance of posture, especially at proximal joints, may well account for many of the signs observed in these patients; the importance of muscle hypotonia in this respect cannot, however, be overlooked. Whether the incoordination and asynergia typical of cerebellar dysfunction reflect only factors such as these, or an additional, perhaps unrelated, deficit is unclear. In any case, from the purely clinical point of view a lesion of the cerebellum or its connections results most importantly in *impairment of coordination,* and the majority of signs encountered in such patients may be interpreted as expressions of this deficit. Such signs, it should be stressed, are ipsilateral to the lesion when the hemispheres are affected.

A characteristic sign of cerebellar disease is *asynergia,* or dysynergia. This consists of an inability to perform movements smoothly because of the lack of normal coordination of agonists, antagonists, and synergists, which results in a jerky and uncoordinated pattern of motility, often referred to as *decomposition of movement.* The incoordination of cerebellar disease, unlike posterior column ataxia, bears no relation to vision and is generally unaffected by eye closure or degree of illumination. More importantly, cerebellar asynergia is not associated with sensory deficits; the disturbance of position sense typical of posterior column (i.e., sensory) ataxia is not found in cerebellar disease. The manner of reaching for and attaining a goal also differs substantially in these two forms of ataxia. Thus, the patient with cerebellar dysfunction tends to utilize accessory muscles in attempting to reach a goal; the limbs often pursue a wide, often random, arc as a result. When placing the finger on the nose, for example, the patient with cerebellar disease will describe a wide trajectory with the arm and will with much jerking and tremor approach and finally reach the nose; in contrast, a patient with posterior column ataxia passes beyond the goal (dysmetria) without these accessory movements. Cerebellar dysynergia is also well displayed in the gait, which is typically ataxic in quality: it is performed on a wide base, the trunk and head held stiffly, the legs extended out from the hips, and the arms flailing about without relation to movement of the legs. The patient lurches and reels and finds it impossible to walk on a narrow base. When dysynergia involves the arms, the affected limbs in addition tend to drift outward when extended against gravity. With specific testing, there is a breakdown of the rate, range, and rhythm of movement as tested by patting, by rapid alternating movements such as pronation/supination, and by tests of manual dexterity.

Asynergia of the musculature of the pharynx and larynx probably accounts for the abnormality of speech found with cerebellar disease. Such speech is slow and hesitant, often scanning, and at times so dysarthric as to be virtually unintelligible. Subtle speech disturbances tend to appear as an early, often overlooked sign of cerebellar disease. Many patients with cerebellar disease also exhibit *hypotonia* of the muscles and a resultant hypermotility of the joints; this is not a consistent feature and is most evident in acutely evolving instances of disease. As noted above, it has been suggested that hypotonia may in fact underlie most if not all of the other clinical manifestations of cerebellar disease.

A delay in starting and stopping movements, expressed as *excessive rebound,* is often noted in patients with cerebellar disease. It is demonstrated most simply by having the patient pull against resistance; with sudden release the limb rebounds to excess without normal checking, and the patient as a result often strikes himself. The same phenomenon can be demonstrated by suddenly depressing the extended arms; a pendular response ensues. Excessive rebound undoubtedly results from faulty postural fixation of the limbs; the same mechanism in all likelihood accounts for the *pendular reflexes,* best demonstrated with the patellar reflexes. The typical cerebellar *intention tremor* is also explicable on this basis.

Cerebellar signs are easily recognized when pronounced but require experience to evaluate in minor degrees. In many instances they are readily identified by the elicitation of asynergia, by observation of the typical gait abnormality, and by notation of intention tremor, of hypotonia, of dysarthria, and of excessive rebound, among others. Not all these signs need be present in all cases, however. For example, severe tremor may on occasion be present with little or no asynergia, or asynergia may be found with only minimal tremor. It is also essential to recognize that cerebellar signs may involve the trunk without involvement of the limbs, or vice versa. As in the cerebral cortex, so too in the cerebellar cortex a pattern of somatotopic localization can be defined (Fig. 3-8); focal lesions will give rise to affection of the trunk or of the limbs, depending on their exact location. The trunk appears to be represented in the midline (vermis), especially superiorly, the limbs more laterally in the hemisphere; the legs seem to be represented anteriorly and superiorly, the arms posteriorly and superiorly. As a result, lesions in the vermis are associated with truncal incoordination and ataxia, whereas lesions in the hemispheres give rise predominantly to incoordination of the appropriate (ipsilateral) limbs.

Generally speaking, the symptoms of cerebellar disease are the same regardless of the point of interruption of the cerebellar apparatus, and it

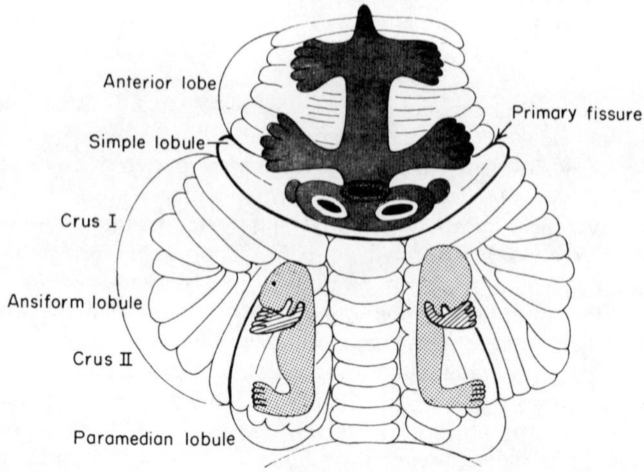


**FIGURE 3-8.** Somatotopic localization in the cerebellar cortex, based on the results of numerous animal studies and confirmed to at least some extent in man. The representation on the superior face (anterior lobe, simple lobule) appears of greatest clinical significance. (Modified from Snider, R. S.: *Interrelations of Cerebellum and Brain Stem.* Res. Publ. Assoc. Res. Nerv. Ment. Dis. 30:267, 1952.)

may not be possible to distinguish affection of the cerebellum itself from that of its pathways and tracts. Tremor, however, tends to be most prominent when there is affection of the superior cerebellar peduncle and becomes increasingly pronounced as the lesion approaches the red nucleus.

### Syndrome of the Vestibular System

Fibers originating in the labyrinth run in the vestibular nerve, itself part of the auditory nerve, and are distributed to the vestibular nuclei in the pontine and medullary tegmentum. Second order connections are made with a host of structures, including anterior horn cells of the spinal cord, cerebellum, oculomotor nuclei via the medial longitudinal fasciculus, and the reticular formation. Disturbances of vestibular function may result from lesions in the labyrinth, the vestibular nerve, the second-order vestibular pathway in the brainstem, the cerebellum, or the cerebrum.

From the symptomatic point of view, interruption of the vestibular system results in *vertigo,* a purely subjective sensation characterized by a disturbance of equilibrium with illusory movement of either the individual (subjective vertigo) or his surroundings (objective vertigo). Nausea and vomiting commonly accompany vertigo, particularly in acute instances. Nystagmus is frequent; it may be horizontal, vertical, or rotary, the last being especially prominent when the lesion involves the labyrinth itself. Vertigo, particularly when of peripheral origin, is commonly precipitated or intensified by rapid changes in posture. Postural changes may also have a substantial effect on the nature and degree of nystagmus. Ataxia or incoordination, especially of the trunk, is often striking with vestibular disease; vestibular ataxia can generally be distinguished from cerebellar ataxia by virtue of the associated vertigo.

## LESIONS INVOLVING SUPERFICIAL SENSATION

Deep sensation has already been dealt with. Disturbances of superficial sensation encountered with lesions at various levels of the nervous system remain to be discussed. Such lesions may involve (1) peripheral nerves; (2) spinal roots; (3) spinal cord; (4) brainstem; (5) thalamus; and (6) cerebral cortex. A more or less distinctive disorder of sensibility can be delineated with lesions in each of these locations (Fig. 3-9).

### Peripheral Nerve Syndrome

The full syndrome of peripheral nerve disease has been discussed (p. 140). In lesions of the peripheral nerve, the sensory disturbances are characterized by a *complete* loss of all forms of sensation (touch, pain, heat, cold, position, vibration) observed in complete interruption of the nerve as occurs, for example, in cases of trauma or of compression; or *partial* loss of sensation in the more common incomplete lesions usually en-

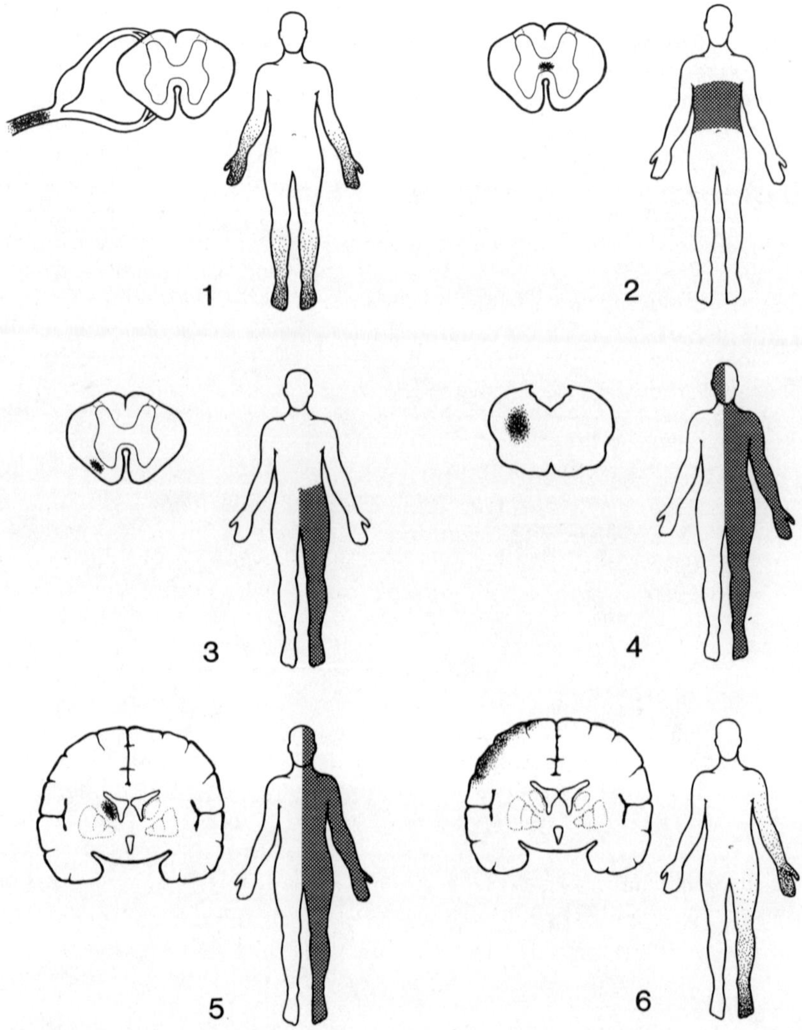


**FIGURE 3-9.** Typical patterns of sensory disturbance with lesions in various parts of the central and peripheral nervous system. *1,* Peripheral nerve(s). *2,* Commissure of spinal cord. *3,* Spinothalamic tract in cord. *4,* Lateral medullary plate. *5,* Thalamus. *6,* Parietal cortex.

countered with metabolic defects, such as diabetes, undernutrition, or porphyria. Such sensory disturbances are found in the distribution of the peripheral nerve or nerves affected. In a typical mononeuropathy, or mononeuritis, the sensory impairment follows a distribution predictable from knowledge of the anatomy of the particular nerve involved. In the more common polyneuropathies, the alteration of sensation tends to assume a symmetrical glove and stocking pattern, which reflects the affection of the distal twigs of a number of sensory nerves. Such a glove and stocking pattern is sometimes confused with the loss of sensation encountered in hysterics. A distinction between the two is based on the following conditions: (1) in polyneuropathy, the impairment of sensation is usually only partial and often does not involve all forms of sensation, whereas in hysteria the sensory defect is typically a complete loss of all modalities; (2) the area of sensory impairment in hysteria is characteristically very sharply defined, whereas in polyneuropathies the transition between area of impairment and area of normalcy is generally indistinct; (3) in polyneuropathy associated features of organic origin (e.g., loss of reflexes) are usually found, whereas this is not the case in hysteria.

Paresthesiae are commonly encountered in disorders of the peripheral nerve, particularly when proprioceptive fibers are involved. Painful dysesthesiae are occasionally observed. Severe pain is sometimes noted, especially in the diabetic and nutritional varieties of polyneuropathy; at times, pain may be sufficiently severe to warrant the use of the term "pseudotabes." When a nerve has been partially damaged but not completely transected, an incapacitating syndrome of intractable pain and dysesthesiae sometimes appears. Known as *causalgia,* this disorder appears to reflect involvement of autonomic fibers within the peripheral nerve.

## Root Syndrome

The posterior roots entering the spinal cord may be involved in a variety of diseases as diverse as tabes dorsalis, herpes zoster, spinal cord tumor, and herniated intervertebral disc, to name but a few. The posterior root syndrome is characterized especially by *pain.* The pain is referred along the specific root (Fig. 3-10). It is severe, constant or intermittent, and typically lancinating in quality. It is usually increased on coughing, straining, sneezing, or with any Valsalva maneuver that increases intraspinal pressure; increase of pain in this fashion probably results from abrupt distention of the subarachnoid sheath surrounding the root, with irritation or compression of the affected root by the fluid wave. While increase with coughing and straining indicates root pain, its absence does not exclude it. Root pain may be so severe as to be unbearable, particularly in cases of acute inflammatory radiculopathy. The terms *radicular pain* and *tabetic pain* are often applied to the pain of root disease.

Sensory impairment is also ordinarily encountered with disease of the posterior spinal roots. This may be in the nature of hyperesthesia (especially in irritative lesions), or loss of superficial sensation (touch, pain, temperature) in the appropriate dermatomal root distribution. Since there is much overlapping of adjacent spinal roots, it is often difficult to map out sensory defects in root disturbances unless more than one root is affected.

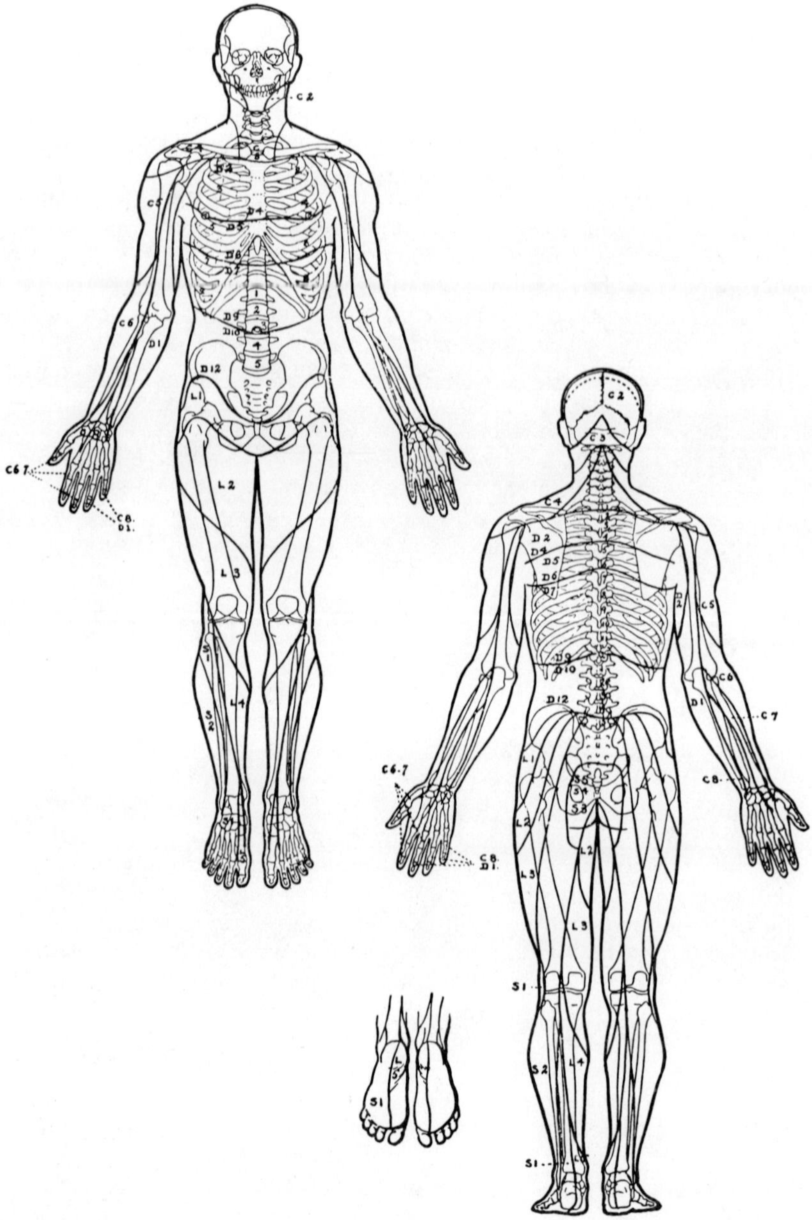


**FIGURE 3-10.** Root sensory skin innervation. A diagrammatic view of the skin areas innervated by the posterior roots.

## Spinal Cord Syndromes

### COMPLETE TRANSVERSE SYNDROME

The syndrome of complete cord transection can be easily recognized. It is found in many conditions, including trauma, spinal cord tumor, transverse myelitis, multiple sclerosis, acute disseminated encephalomyelitis, and meningovascular syphilis. It is characterized by the following:

**PARALYSIS.** *Paralysis* below the level of the lesion is seen. Early in the course, this is flaccid and areflexic; spasticity and hyperreflexia develop with the passage of time.

**LOSS OF SENSATION.** Complete *loss of all modalities of sensation* below the level of the lesion is found. In some circumstances, and especially with extramedullary cord tumors, a zone of hyperesthesia can be identified at the top of the sensory level.

**SPHINCTER DISTURBANCES.** There is retention of urine in acute cases, which in the course of a few days or weeks evolves into automatic emptying. Fecal incontinence is also found.

**TROPHIC DISTURBANCES.** Atrophy and trophic ulcers of the skin appear, along with disturbances of the nails in the paralyzed segments. A loss of sweating is generally found below the level of the lesion.

As already pointed out, the manifestations of transverse lesions of the spinal cord vary with the rapidity of development of the process. In acutely developing transverse sections (e.g., in cord injuries and transverse myelitis) the clinical features are those of *spinal shock.* The paralyzed muscles are flaccid, the reflexes are lost, there is complete sensory loss below the level of the lesion, and retention of urine and feces is found. This stage may last 3 weeks or longer and is followed by recovery of reflex activity which is manifested by a return of flexor reflexes in response to noxious stimuli applied to the skin. At times a *mass reflex* is encountered. This comprises flexor spasms of the legs and lower abdominal wall, evacuation of the bladder, and profuse sweating. Tendon reflexes return during this stage and are exaggerated. Reflex emptying of the bladder and bowel may also appear at this time. With more gradually evolving transverse lesions such as intramedullary tumor, spinal shock is not encountered. The legs become weak and spastic and eventually completely paralyzed if the process is not relieved. Weakness usually develops before sensory loss in cases of compression from without, as in extramedullary tumors, since motor fibers appear to be more susceptible than sensory to such injury. Gradually, however, sensory impairment also ensues. Alterations in sphincter control generally parallel the appearance of pyramidal tract signs. The final result is the typical transverse syndrome characterized by spastic paraplegia, sensory loss, and sphincter abnormalities.

## BROWN-SÉQUARD SYNDROME

In its purest form, this is found in instances of hemisection of the spinal cord. It results from either intramedullary or extramedullary lesions and is perhaps most commonly seen in instances of cord trauma. Paralysis, loss of position and vibration senses, and ataxia (sensory ataxia) are encountered on the side of the lesion and reflect involvement of the corticospinal pathway and the posterior column. Contralateral to the lesion, loss of pain and temperature senses is found as a result of affection of the spinothalamic tract. At times, a narrow band of impairment of such superficial sensation is also encountered ipsilaterally, at the segmental level of the lesion itself; this is, however, very difficult to demonstrate.

The Brown-Séquard syndrome is, as often as not, encountered in a less than complete, or classic, form. It often presents in an incomplete manner, for example, with loss of pain and temperature sense on the opposite side of the body below the level of the lesion, with but few ipsilateral signs.

## COMMISSURAL SYNDROME

This is the result of a lesion involving the central gray matter of the spinal cord. It is found particularly in syringomyelia, but may also be encountered in instances of trauma with hematomyelia and in cases of spinal cord tumor, among others. It is characterized by loss of pain and temperature sensations due to interruption of these fibers as they cross from the posterior horns to the spinothalamic tract. Other sensory modalities are spared. The sensory loss is bilateral, since fibers from both sides must inevitably be interrupted in such a lesion, and segmental, in that it involves only the fibers of the segments involved. Thus, a lesion that involves the central gray matter of segments T2-T5 will produce loss of pain and temperature sensation restricted to these segments. The commissural syndrome can be produced only by a lesion within the cord substance; it is anatomically impossible for an extramedullary lesion to elicit this disorder of sensibility.

## SPINOTHALAMIC TRACT SYNDROME

A lesion involving the spinothalamic tract in the anterolateral portion of the spinal cord results in a loss of pain and temperature sensations on the opposite side of the body, affecting all the segments below the level of the lesion. Pain and temperature sensations may not be impaired with equal severity; one, usually pain, may be affected more than the other. The

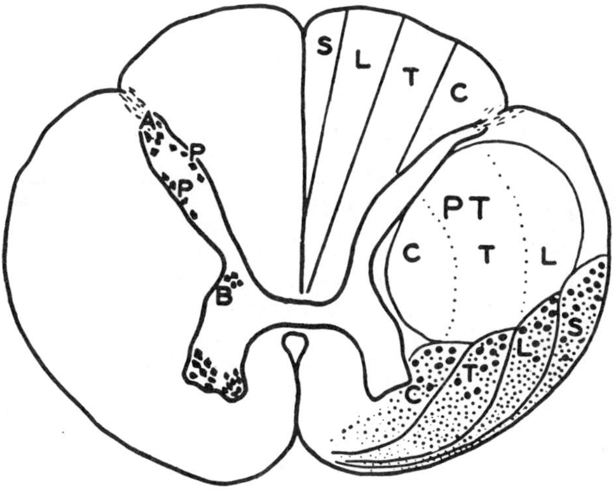


**FIGURE 3-11.** Diagrammatic representation of distribution of fibers in the spinothalamic tract in the spinal cord. The sacral fibers are most laterally placed, the cervical most medially. The reverse pattern of lamellation may be noted in the posterior columns.

term "dissociated" is sometimes applied to this pattern of sensory defect, in that certain modalities (pain, temperature) are involved, whereas others (in this instance, posterior column modalities such as position and vibration sense) are spared. Numerous intramedullary and extramedullary processes may give rise to the syndrome. Within the spinothalamic tract, it should be noted, the fibers are arranged in laminar fashion: the sacral fibers are located at the periphery, fibers from higher levels more centrally (Fig. 3-11). Hence, an intramedullary process will often involve the fibers from the more superior levels first and may spare the more peripheral sacral fibers. This results in a phenomenon referred to as *sacral sparing,* which implies preservation of sensation in the sacral segments (e.g., saddle area) with impairment of sensation at other and higher segmental levels. Sacral sparing is commonly although not invariably associated with intramedullary disease, particularly expanding lesions such as an intramedullary glioma. Extramedullary lesions, on the other hand, compress the cord from without and result in involvement of the sacral fibers as well as those from higher levels. It will incidentally be noted that a reverse lamellation obtains in the posterior columns, where the lumbar and sacral fibers are found most deeply, the cervical most laterally. This is, however, of relatively minor clinical significance.

## POSTERIOR HORN SYNDROME

Ipsilateral impairment of pain and temperature may be found with affection of the fibers subserving these sensory modalities at the base of the posterior horn before they decussate in the commissure. This is usually the result of a syringomyelic cavity. The resulting sensory disturbance may extend for a variable number of segments. Posterior column modalities (position, vibration sense) typically escape. If the lesion extends into the root entry zone, radicular pain may appear.

### POSTEROLATERAL SYNDROME

Many lesions involve more or less selectively the posterior and lateral columns of the cord, for example, subacute combined degeneration of the cord with pernicious anemia, and Friedreich's ataxia. Other less systematized disorders such as multiple sclerosis may produce much the same deficit. The syndrome consists of impairment or loss of those sensory modalities that traverse the posterior columns, that is, position and vibration senses, but with preservation of pain and temperature sensibility, since the spinothalamic tracts are not involved. Typically, pyramidal tract signs (weakness, spasticity, hyperreflexia, extensor plantar responses) accompany the sensory affection. By virtue of the loss of proprioception, rombergism is prominent, along with sensory ataxia.

## Medullary Syndrome

When a lesion involves the lateral tegmentum of the medulla, as in infarction in the distribution of the posterior inferior cerebellar artery (Wallenberg's syndrome), a highly typical pattern of sensory impairment is observed. There is loss of pain and temperature sense on the opposite side of the body, reflecting affection of the spinothalamic fibers at this level. In addition, however, one generally encounters impairment of these modalities over the face, but in an ipsilateral distribution, due to involvement of the spinal tract and nucleus of the trigeminal nerve. The result, therefore, is a very characteristic crossed sensory loss. Ordinarily, other clinical manifestations such as ipsilateral cerebellar ataxia, hoarseness, dysphagia, and a Horner's syndrome accompany the defect. Above the medulla, on the other hand, all sensory fibers, whether derived from the body or from the face, run together, since the fibers originating in the trigeminal nerve decussate and assume a position in the quintothalamic tract, closely applied to the spinothalamic tract itself. As a result, lesions in the brainstem above the medulla tend to produce impairment of pain and temperature sense on the opposite side of the face as well as of the body.

## Thalamic Syndrome

Since the thalamus is the end station of all crude forms of sensibility, a complete lesion that involves the sensory nuclei of the thalamus results in impairment or loss of all forms of sensation on the opposite side of the face, trunk, and limbs, along with a variable motor defect. Astereognosis is often found, presumably a reflection of the impairment of proprioception. Many patients so afflicted experience pain, which may be deep, paroxysmal, and excruciating in nature, or at times constant, burning, and causalgia-like. Such pain may involve the entire opposite side of the body, or only a portion thereof. In addition to the spontaneous pain, a variety of relatively minor stimuli will cause unpleasant sensations (dysesthesiae), often with radiation of the sensation beyond the point of stimulation. The combination of sensory impairment, spontaneous pain, and perversion of cutaneous sensibility, or dysesthesiae, is sometimes referred to as the *thalamic syndrome* of Déjérine-Roussy. The impairment of sensation may be relatively mild as compared with the degree of spontaneous pain of which the patient complains.

## Cortical Syndrome

Sensory disturbances caused by involvement of the sensory (parietal) cortex are not as sharply defined as in lesions that implicate lower levels. Discriminatory sensations are more severely affected than superficial or crude sensations. In general, one observes: (1) Loss of position sense, with little or no impairment of vibration sense. (2) Absence of involvement of other crude forms of sensation, such as pain, touch, and temperature. This is not an absolute rule, however, and pain sensibility may be decreased, particularly in the distal portions of the contralateral limbs. Touch, heat, and cold are not usually affected. Impairment of these crude modalities tends to appear when the deeper parietal white matter is involved, that is, when the lesion is close to the thalamus, and is much less in evidence when the lesion is relatively confined to the cortical mantle itself. (3) Impairment of discrimination, that is, of so-called cortical sensibility, for example, detection of the two points of a compass, appreciation of differences in texture or weight, and recognition of figures written on the skin (agraphaesthesia). (4) Astereognosis, or the inability to identify the shape or nature of objects placed in the hand. Stereognosis is dependent upon the ability to recognize size, shape, weight, texture, and other physical attributes of objects and represents a synthesis of these individual characteristics into a meaningful whole (Gestalt). A loss of this ability is called astereognosis, or tactile agnosia. It is commonly regarded as dependent upon sensory disturbance, particularly loss of touch and proprioception; on the other hand, some restrict the use of the term to those cases in which sensation is intact. (5) Sensory jacksonian seizures. (6) Rarely, spontaneous pain.

In addition to these sensory difficulties, when a rapidly evolving lesion such as a softening involves the minor (nondominant, usually right) parietal lobe, disturbances of the body scheme appear (see above). There is disagreement as to whether the body image, or body scheme, is in fact localized to the nondominant parietal lobe, or whether it is bilaterally represented. According to the latter view, the presence of language disorders (aphasia) with dominant hemisphere lesions precludes evaluation of the body image in the majority of cases and leads to an erroneous impression of lateralization of function.

## LESIONS OF THE SPHINCTERS

Loss of sphincter control occurs under many circumstances in the human. The problem is complex, and a review of the normal control of the sphincters is pertinent. Recognition of the functional and pharmacologic interrelationships of the bladder innervation is essential to an understanding of derangements of bladder function, and to their management. Disturbances of micturition are, it should be stressed, of greater practical significance than those of defecation, since they are much more frequently encountered in neurologic disease.

### Bladder

Micturition is a function of the peripheral autonomic nervous system and is subject to control from higher centers in the brainstem, basal ganglia, and cerebrum. The bladder empties by means of a reciprocal action of its involuntary smooth musculature, the detrusor and the internal sphincter (Fig. 3-12). These receive their innervation from the hypogastric nerve (T-11, 12, L-1), which is derived from the lumbar sympathetic chain and is, thus, adrenergic in type, and from the pelvic nerve (S-2, 3, 4), which represents the cholinergic parasympathetic innervation via the sacral plexus. The striated external sphincter muscle and the voluntary muscles of the perineum are innervated by the pudendal nerves (S-2, 3, 4).

Both alpha and beta adrenergic receptors can be identified in the bladder. Alpha receptors are found predominantly at the base of the bladder, that is, at the trigone and the inferior part of the detrusor, and alpha adrenergic stimulation induces contraction of the smooth muscles there. Beta receptors characterize the body of the bladder, that is, the bulk of the detrusor; as anticipated, beta stimulation results in detrusor relaxation. Cholinergic stimulation, on the other hand, results in bladder (detrusor) contraction, a response only partially blocked by atropine. Electrophysiologic studies yield complementary results. Thus, stimulation of the peripheral segment of the cut pelvic nerves in animals causes powerful contraction of the detrusor muscle with relaxation of the internal sphincter. Stimulation of the hypogastric nerves causes contraction of the internal sphincter in animals and man, accompanied by inhibition of action of the detrusor. Stimulation of the pudendal nerve causes contraction of the external sphincter. The integrity of the pelvic nerves is of paramount importance for normal micturition; section of these nerves causes profound suppression of micturition with an atonic distended bladder. Section of the hypogastric, pelvic, and pudendal nerves is followed, after a

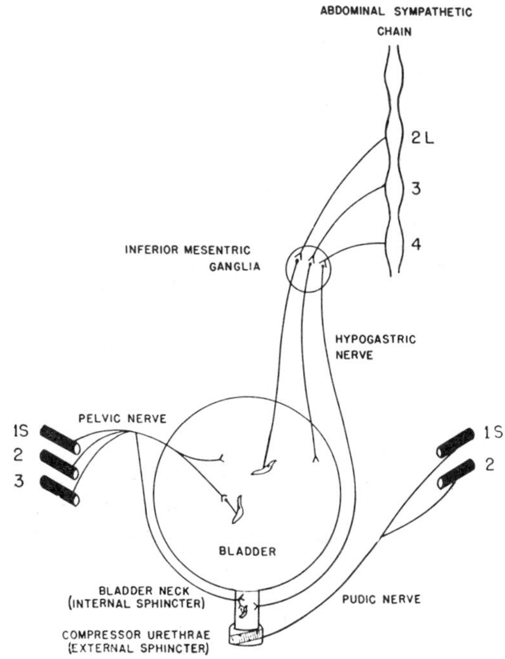


**FIGURE 3-12.** Innervations of bladder, showing the central and peripheral innervations of the detrusor, and the internal and external sphincters. (From Learmonth and McLeod: *Physiology in Modern Medicine.* ed. 9. C. V. Mosby Co., p. 1128.)

short period of retention, by periodic discharge or automatic micturition.

The parasympathetic center for micturition in the spinal cord is found in segments S-2 and 3; the sympathetic center lies in the lumbar cord. These spinal centers are under the control of supraspinal centers located in the pons and midbrain, which are in turn themselves subject to the influence of still higher centers in the cerebral hemispheres, and perhaps in the basal ganglia. Cerebral control of the bladder seems to be inhibitory in function. The cortical area responsible for bladder control lies near the leg area of the motor cortex; in man, bilateral lesions of the paracentral lobule, as encountered, for example, with parasagittal meningiomas or in instances of bilateral anterior cerebral artery occlusion, result in incontinence. The incontinence noted in patients with normal pressure hydrocephalus is thought to reflect stretching of the nerve fibers derived from the paracentral lobule in their course around the enlarged ventricles that are characteristic of the disease.

The normal act of micturition reflects these functional properties. Micturition is essentially dependent on a stretch reflex acting on the detrusor muscle; the stimulus is the stretch evoked by the increasing volume of the bladder contents and by the resultant rise in intravesical pressure. As a result of distention of the bladder, afferent impulses in the pelvic nerve reach the spinal cord and a multisynaptic reflex arc is established, which rises at least as high as the brainstem. As a result of descending impulses traveling primarily in the lateral, ventral, and medial reticulospinal pathways, detrusor contraction is initiated via impulses conveyed through the pelvic nerve; the segmental reflex is mediated at the S-2, 3, 4 level. When the detrusor contracts, reciprocal relaxation of the sphincters follows.

## TYPES OF BLADDER DISTURBANCE

Two principle forms of disordered bladder function are found in the human; they are commonly designated *atonic* and *hyportonic* (or, in the terminology of Krane and Siroky, *detrusor areflexia* or *hyporeflexia,* and *detrusor hyperreflexia).* In the past, the terms "neurogenic" and "cord" bladder were used to designate bladder disturbances of peripheral or central nervous system origin, respectively. Such terms are confusing, however, and lack precision; whenever possible the exact form of bladder dysfunction in a physiologic sense should be defined. The use of a multitude of other obscure terms that have found favor from time to time is also to be discouraged. The term "autonomous bladder" has sometimes been used to designate an abnormality of bladder function secondary to a lesion distal to the sacral cord itself, that is, a denervated bladder. Synonymous terms include "lower motor neuron bladder," "sensory paralytic bladder," "motor paralytic bladder," and "autonomous neurogenic bladder"; all these are more accurately incorporated in the contemporary rubric of detrusor hyporeflexia, or atonic bladder. The term "reflex bladder" has at times been used to imply a hypertonic bladder, currently understood as detrusor hyperreflexia; other inexact designations that have been so used include "automatic bladder," "upper motor neuron bladder," "reflex neurogenic bladder," and "uninhibited neurogenic bladder." The plethora of terms underscores the need for clarification and simplification.

The atonic bladder, that is, the bladder characterized by detrusor hyporeflexia, is found with lesions of the sacral segments of the spinal cord (conus medullaris) and in disease of the cauda equina and of the pelvic nerves. It is characterized by loss of tone of the detrusor muscle with urinary retention and increased bladder capacity along with loss of sensation associated with bladder distention. The patient is generally unable to tell when the bladder is full. Under such circumstances, the bladder tends to become extremely distended, but without a sensation of fullness or discomfort. Automatic emptying follows. The urine is usually discharged in small quantities and the bladder is incompletely emptied. The cystometrogram demonstrates increased bladder capacity, with a very slow rise in vesical pressure during filling, and an ability to retain a large amount of fluid before sufficient stretch is produced to cause reflex contraction.

An atonic bladder response also appears in lesions that involve the posterior roots, which interfere with the afferent portion of the reflex arc. Deafferentation of this sort occurs in striking fashion in tabes dorsalis, but is also encountered in diabetes and, at times, in other metabolic polyneuropathies. Under these circumstances, the bladder capacity is also greatly increased, there is no sensation of distention of the bladder, detrusor tone is lost, and there is incontinence caused by relaxation of the internal sphincter and impaired detrusor action. Emptying the bladder is possible by normal volition, but the stream is feeble and residual urine is always found.

In brief, then, the atonic bladder results essentially from interruption of either the afferent or efferent peripheral pathways to the bladder, or both. In contrast is the hypertonic bladder, that is, the bladder characterized by detrusor hyperreflexia, which results from affection of the autonomic pathways above the level of the sacral outflow. This may result from bilateral lesions of the spinal cord above the sacral segments, or from bilateral involvement of the motor cortex or of the pyramidal tract anywhere in its course. In the hypertonic bladder, capacity is reduced. The vesical pressure rises rapidly during filling, so that relatively little urine can collect before the desire for micturition develops. Urgency and frequency are thus characteristic symptoms. Unlike the atonic bladder, sensation is not lost, and bladder distention is associated with a feeling of discomfort. The bladder is emptied completely with each act of urination. Depending upon the exact site of the responsible lesion, there may be a loss of the normal functional inter-relationship between the detrusor muscle on the one hand and the external sphincter on the other. This phenomenon, referred to as *vesicosphincter dysynergia,* may reflect release of a facilitative reflex. It appears with lesions above the sacral segments of the spinal cord, but below the pons. When the lesion is above the pons, such dysynergia does not occur.

In instances of complete transection of the cord above the sacral segments, an *automatic bladder* may become established. Following the stage of flaccid paralysis and distention of the bladder, automatic contraction of the bladder wall develops with expulsion of urine but without complete emptying. At times, the automatic emptying is part of the mass reflex described previously. Automatic bladder function may develop in 4 to 5 weeks after cord transection, but in many instances may take up to 6 months or longer to appear, and in some individuals it never develops.

As indicated above, Krane and Siroky, emphasizing the functional characteristics of the defects, propose a classification of bladder disorders centering about the principle categories of detrusor hyperreflexia and detrusor areflexia.

*Detrusor hyperreflexia* may be subdivided into three types. (1) A form with *coordinated* sphincters exhibiting the anticipated appropriate relaxation of the sphincters with detrusor contraction may be observed. Such coordinated action is dependent upon the integrity of the descending tracts from the pons that subserve detrusor-sphincter coordination.

Lesions above the pons (i.e., in the cerebrum or basal ganglia), as in dementing processes, or with cerebrovascular disease or parkinsonism, appear responsible; at times, incomplete cord lesions are found. (2) When lesions involve the descending pathways below the level of the pons, *vesicosphincter dysynergia* involving the external (striated) sphincter appears and is commonly associated with incontinence. Myelopathies such as transverse myelitis or spinal cord trauma are often implicated. (3) When the responsible lesion involves the upper portion of the spinal cord, that is, the upper thoracic and cervical segments, dysynergia of the smooth muscle sphincter may also appear.

Several subtypes of *detrusor areflexia* may also be recognized. (1) A form with coordinated detrusor-sphincter action results from partial bladder denervation; the lesion is either central (sacral) or peripheral. (2) Under similar circumstances, a variety characterized by failure of relaxation of the external sphincter is occasionally encountered. (3) Following extensive pelvic surgery with damage to both the parasympathetic and pudendal outflow, or with lesions of the cauda equina, denervation of the external sphincter may accompany the detrusor areflexia. (4) Finally, a form of detrusor areflexia is recognized in which nonrelaxation of the smooth muscle sphincter reflects interference with parasympathetic innervation.

Recognition of such pathophysiologic mechanisms fosters a rational approach to management of patients with disorders of bladder function. In brief, pharmacologic manipulation of detrusor hyperreflexia (spasticity) is based on the use of anticholinergic agents, for example, Pro-Banthine, along with direct smooth muscle relaxants such as oxybutynin (Ditropan). Therapy of detrusor hyporeflexia, on the other hand, is based on the use of cholinergic agents such as bethanechol (Urecholine); alpha adrenergic blockers, such as phenoxybenzamine; and direct smooth muscle relaxants with cholinergic properties, such as oxybutynin. Adrenergic agents, for example, imipramine (Tofranil), may play a role in the treatment of enuresis by virtue of their ability to increase bladder capacity. Striated muscle relaxants such as baclofen or diazepam may be of assistance in instances of external sphincter spasm.

Finally, it should be emphasized that many of these disorders may be mimicked by non-neurologic lesions or by psychogenic disorders. Thorough investigations utilizing not only cystometrograms but also sphincter electromyography and rapid pharmacologic testing are essential for an accurate pathogenetic formulation in any given case.

## Rectum

The normal act of defecation is characterized by contraction of the rectum and reciprocal relaxation of the anal sphincter. The adequate stimulus is tension on the wall of the rectum, which brings about a stretch reflex and contraction of the rectum. The reciprocal relationship between rectum and internal sphincter is nervous in mechanism and is mediated solely through the lower sacral segments of the spinal cord (S2, 3, 4) and its peripheral plexuses. Destruction of the sacral segments of the spinal cord or its roots results in relaxation of the sphincter and continuous bowel evacuation; a lax anal sphincter, loss of sensation of bowel fullness, and fecal incontinence are observed clinically. A lesion of the spinal cord above the sacral segments generally results in constipation, at times with intermittent involuntary emptying of the bowel.

## Sexual Function

Sexual function in the male is extremely complex and reflects both neural and psychic influences. As with bladder innervation, the anatomic mechanisms underlying particularly male sexual function include both parasympathetic and sympathetic components; the final pathway is adrenergic in type. Parasympathetic fibers originate in sacral segments 2, 3, and 4 and run in the pelvic nerve to the corpora cavernosa. Stimulation results in erection; damage to the parasympathetic innervation as, for example, following radical prostatectomy or abdominoperoneal resection, frequently leads to impotence. Sympathetic fibers run in the hypogastric nerve and are derived from T12-L4; they innervate the vasa deferentia, the seminal vesicles, and the posterior urethra, as well as the penile vasculature. Some role in erection is also postulated for these fibers; sympathectomy not uncommonly results in impotence. Somatic innervation to the bulbocavernosus, ischiocavernosus, and external urethral sphincter originates in the sacral cord (S2, 3, 4) and travels in the pudendal nerve; this nerve also provides sensory supply to the skin of the penis. Lesions of the spinal cord or of the peripheral autonomic nervous system may interfere with these normal neural patterns and result in impotence. Thus, diabetics with autonomic neuropathy or patients on chronic hemodialysis with uremic neuropathy are commonly impotent. Affection of the posterior spinal roots, as in tabes, or of the cord parenchyma itself, seen in cord tumor, multiple sclerosis, or synringomyelia, among others, may similarly produce impotence. With high cord lesions reflex erection may occur, although there is no response to psychogenic stimulation; at times, persistent, often painful erection (priapism) is observed under such circumstances.

From the pharmacologic point of view, ganglionic blocking agents such as atropine or Pro-Banthine may cause impotence, as will beta adrenergic blockers. Alpha adrenergic blockers, on the other hand, rarely affect erection, although they have a distinct effect on ejaculation.

Organic lesions of the cerebral hemispheres that involve especially the primitive rhinencephalic/limbic portions of the brain may similarly cause impotence or other changes in sexual function. Patients with temporal lobe epilepsy are often impotent, as are individuals with damage to the temporal lobes after a severe head injury. Alteration of sexual function is a prominent characteristic of the Klüver-Bucy syndrome, as seen experimentally following bilateral temporal lobectomy, and occasionally reproduced in humans. Impotence is also a frequent symptom in disorders that involve the substantia nigra, such as parkinsonism and the Shy-Drager syndrome. Finally, of course, the remarkable influence of psychogenic factors on both potency and libido should not be underestimated; such psychic influences may, in fact, be mediated via the medial temporal (hippocampal) structures.

Little is known concerning sexual function in the female in the face of neurologic disease. Heightened sexual activity has been described with lesions of the limbic lobe, and a loss of sexual sensation may be encountered in diseases of the cauda equina or peripheral nerves. Parasympathetic stimulation is known to result in increased vaginal secretion and clitoral erection. For the most part, however, alteration of female sexual function provides little assistance in achieving an accurate topical diagnosis of neurologic disease.

## BIBLIOGRAPHY


Albert, M., Goodglass, H., Helm, N., Rubins, A., et al.: *Clinical Aspects of Dysphasia.* Springer-Verlag, Berlin (in press).

Appenzeller, O.: *The Autonomic Nervous System.* North Holland Publishing, Amsterdam, 1976.

Benson, D. F.: Aphasia, Alexia, and Agraphia. Churchill Livingstone, New York, 1979.

Bradley, W. E., Rockswold, G. L., Timm, G. W., et al.: *Neurology of micturition.* J. Urol. 115:481, 1976.

Brain, L.: *Speech Disorders: Aphasia, Apraxia, and Agnosia.* Butterworths, Washington, 1965.

Brock, S. A.: *Basis of Clinical Neurology.* ed. 4. Williams & Wilkins, Baltimore, 1963.

Chadwick, D., Reynolds, E. H., and Marsden, C. D.: *Anticonvulsant-induced dyskinesias: a comparison with dyskinesias induced by neuroleptics.* J. Neurol. Neurosurg. Psychiatry 39:1210, 1976.

Chambers, W. W., and Sprague, J. M.: *Functional localization in the cerebellum. II. Somatotopic organization of cortex and nuclei.* Arch. Neurol. Psychiatry 74:6, 1955.

Chapman, L. F., and Wolff, H. G.: *Cerebral hemispheres and highest integrative functions of man.* Arch. Neurol. Psychiatry 1:357, 1959.

Cogan, D.: *Neurology of the Ocular Muscles.* ed. 2. Charles C Thomas, Springfield, Ill., 1963.

Cogan, D. G.: *Neurology of the Visual System.* Charles C Thomas, Springfield, Ill., 1966.

Critchely, M.: *The Parietal Lobes.* Hafner Publishing, New York, 1953.

Critchley, M.: *Developmental Dyslexia.* William Heinemann, London, 1964.

Darley, F. L., and Millikan, C. H. (eds.): *Brain Mechanisms Underlying Speech and Language.* Grune & Stratton, New York, 1967.

Denny-Brown, D.: *Diseases of the basal ganglia: their relation to disorders of movement.* Lancet 2:1099–1155, 1960.

Dow, R. S., and Moruzzi, G.: *The Physiology and Pathology of the Cerebellum.* University of Minnesota Press, Minneapolis, 1958.

Eldridge, R., and Fahn, S. (eds.): *Dystonia. Advances in Neurology.* vol. 14. Raven Press, New York, 1976.

Ettlinger, E. G., deReuck, A. V. S., and Porter, R. (eds.): *Functions of the Corpus Callosum.* Ciba Foundation Study Group No. 20. Little, Brown and Co., Boston, 1965.

Geschwind, N.: *Disconnexion syndromes in animals and man.* Brain 88: 237, 585, 1965.

Geschwind, N.: "The clinical syndromes of the cortical connections." In Williams, D. (ed.): *Modern Trends in Neurology.* Butterworths, London, 1970, Chapter 2.

Geschwind, N.: *Aphasia.* N. Engl. J. Med. 284:654, 1971.

Goldstein, K.: *Language and Language Disturbances.* Grune & Stratton, New York, 1948.

Harrington, D. O.: *The Visual Fields.* ed. 3. C. V. Mosby Company, St. Louis, 1971.

Head, H.: *Aphasia and Kindred Disorders of Speech.* Macmillan Co., New York, 1926.

Krane, R. J., and Siroky, M. B.: *Clinical Neuro-Urology.* Little, Brown and Co., Boston, 1979.

Luria, A. R.: *Human Brain and Psychological Processes.* Harper & Row, New York, 1966.

Magoun, H., and Rhines, R.: *Spasticity.* Charles C Thomas. Springfield, Ill., 1947.

Marsden, C. D.: "Dystonia: the spectrum of the disease." In Yahr, M. D. (ed.): *The Basal Ganglia.* Raven Press, New York, 1976.

Nielson, J. M.: *Agnosia, Apraxia, Aphasia: Their Value in Cerebral Localization.* Paul B. Hoeber, New York, 1946.

Northern, J. (ed.): *Hearing Disorders.* Little, Brown & Co., Boston, 1976.

Penfield, W.: *The cerebral cortex in man. I. The cerebral cortex and consciousness.* Arch. Neurol. Psychiatry 40:417, 1938.

Rioch, D. McK., and Weinstein, E. A. (eds.): *Disorders of communication.* Res. Publ. Assoc. Res. Nerv. Ment. Dis. vol. 42, 1964.

Simpson, G. M., and Kline, N. S.: "Tardive dyskinesia: manifestations, incidence, etiology, and treatment. In Yahr, M. D. (ed.): *The Basal Ganglia.* Raven Press, New York, 1976.

Walshe, F. M. R.: *Critical Studies in Neurology.* Williams & Wilkins, Baltimore, 1948.

Wiesenburg, T., and McBride, K. E.: *Aphasia: A Clinical and Psychological Study (1935).* Hafner Publishing, New York, 1964 (reprint).

Wepman, J. M., and Jones, L. F.: *Five aphasias: a commentary on aphasia as a regressive linguistic phenomenon.* Res. Publ. Assoc. Res. Nerv. Ment. Dis. 42:190, 1964.
Whitaker, H., and Whitaker H. (eds.): *Perspectives in Neurolinguistics and Psycholinguistics.* vol. 1. Academic Press, New York, 1976.

# 4

# LABORATORY INVESTIGATIONS IN NEUROLOGIC DISEASE

A variety of special examinations that supplement careful clinical appraisal is often required in the evaluation of patients with disease of the nervous system. Brief consideration of some of the more common techniques employed, and of the indications for their use, is therefore appropriate here.

## LUMBAR PUNCTURE

Lumbar puncture, providing for detailed examination of the cerebrospinal fluid, represents in many ways the simplest and one of the most informative of the ancillary tests available to the clinical neurologist. It should be performed only with the greatest caution in the presence of increased intracranial pressure, and it is particularly hazardous in instances of expanding lesions in the posterior fossa. The risk of herniation of the brain under pressure through either the free edge of the tentorium (uncal herniation) or foramen magnum (cerebellar tonsillar herniation) should not be underestimated under these circumstances; even if only a small amount of spinal fluid is removed at the time of the tap, continued leakage of fluid through the puncture wound in the meninges may lead to delayed herniation. In general, lumbar puncture should be carried out in the face of an increase in intracranial pressure only when necessary for diagnostic purposes, for example, when the possibility of purulent or granulomatous meningitis must be excluded, and then only with full knowledge of the risks being undertaken. In the last analysis, of course, a lumbar puncture is indicated whenever information derived from examination of the cerebrospinal fluid is deemed essential for effective patient management.

In considering the mechanical aspects of the procedure, proper positioning of the patient is indispensable. The patient is placed on his side, with the head and body acutely flexed, and the knees drawn up on the abdomen and clasped firmly by the hands. The back is prepared with cutaneous antiseptics and draped with sterile towels. The puncture itself is performed under aseptic precautions, utilizing a needle as fine as consistent with accurate pressure readings. The tap is best carried out between the fourth and fifth or third and fourth lumbar vertebrae, the latter being preferred because of frequent anomalies that involve the former. Palpation of the iliac crest provides a useful landmark, since it ordinarily lies opposite the fourth lumbar vertebra. Procaine is injected into the skin as a local anesthetic; it is not necessary to anesthetize the subcutaneous and muscle tissues. The lumbar puncture needle is inserted in the midline or 1 cm to one side of the midline and is directed slightly upward. Entrance into the subarachnoid space is felt as a "give" before the needle as it penetrates the dura, immediately below which lies the subarachnoid membrane. If the puncture has been performed without trauma, clear fluid is obtained on withdrawal of the stylet. The water manometer for measuring pressure of the spinal fluid should then be attached and the level of the fluid column measured after it has come to rest. The patient must be relaxed to obtain an accurate pressure reading. Repositioning of the head and legs, thus uncoiling the patient to some extent, is advisable before an elevated pressure reading is accepted as meaningful.

In cases of suspected block of the spinal subarachnoid space, a Queckenstedt test may be performed; it is however, not without hazard, and finds little application today. It should never be carried out in instances of disease above the foramen magnum, especially if a mass lesion is suspected. Jugular compression is provided manually, or with a blood pressure cuff. The rise of spinal fluid pressure at the end of 10 seconds is recorded; following the release of compression, the level of pressure is recorded 10 seconds later. In normal individuals, a rapid and high rise of spinal fluid pressure (to 400 or 500 mm of water) follows bilateral jugular compression, with return of pressure to its original level within 10 to 15 seconds after release of the jugular compression. The test is completed by having the patient strain, then cough; a similar rise in pressure occurs. Elevation of intraspinal pressure following compression of the jugular veins reflects an increase in intracranial pressure as a result of interference with venous escape from the skull. If a block is present in the subarachnoid space, no measurable rise, or only an imperfect one, is demonstrable at the lumbar needle with jugular compression. Coughing and straining will elicit a rise in pressure, however, since the increased abdominal pressure prevents escape of blood from the spinal veins. It must be emphasized, however, that with the ready availability of myelography there is little or no indication for this test in contemporary neurologic practice.

After determination of the initial spinal fluid pressure, cerebrospinal fluid (CSF) is removed for routine examination, which includes at the least determination of cell count, protein and sugar content, and tests for syphilis. Special studies, such as microbiologic culture or determination of gamma globulin or myelin basic protein, or a search for cryptococcal antigen, should be undertaken as indicated. The level of spinal fluid pressure is again recorded after the fluid is withdrawn. The spinal fluid, particularly if bloody, should be drawn into several successive tubes. This technique is valuable in the identification of a traumatic tap, since the blood under such circumstances generally disappears by the third tube. Immediate centrifugation of the spinal fluid to look for xanthochromia in the supernatant may also assist in identifying a traumatic puncture.

Following the lumbar puncture, the patient is instructed to lie flat for 8 to 12 hours in an attempt to avoid a post-lumbar puncture headache; the intake of liquids should be encouraged. The appearance of a post-lumbar puncture headache is not a predictable event; it is probably related more to persistent leak of spinal fluid from the arachnoidal puncture site than to factors such as amount of fluid withdrawn, anxiety, or failure to remain recumbent.

## Cistern Puncture

This investigation is required only under exceptional circumstances by virtue of its inherent risks. The patient is placed on his side, the head sharply flexed and rotation of the neck avoided. The puncture site is shaved, prepared with cutaneous antiseptics, and draped with sterile towels. The spine of the second cervical vertebra is identified and the thumb of the examiner's left hand held firmly down on the spine. The needle is then directed along the knuckle of the flexed left thumb, the point coming directly in the center of the depression above the second cervical spine. The needle is then directed in the midline slightly upward along a line transecting the external auditory meatus and the bridge of the nose. After two or three resistances are encountered a sudden "give" is felt, which indicates entrance of the needle into the cisterna magna. This is ordinarily reached in thin-necked persons at a depth of about 4 cm, and in thick-necked individuals at about 5 cm. If blood is encountered the needle should be withdrawn and no further attempt made. If the neck has been in good position and the needle held strictly in the midline in the direction indicated, the cistern will ordinarily be reached without difficulty.

## The Cerebrospinal Fluid

The *normal* spinal fluid pressure as recorded at lumbar puncture utilizing a water manometer varies from 100 to 200 mm. Pressures over 200 mm are definitely elevated, those of 180 to 200 mm are borderline. The cell content of the spinal fluid varies normally from one to four lymphocytes; a white cell content of six cells or more is abnormal. The spinal fluid ordinarily has a protein content of 25 to 45 mg per 100 ml, somewhat higher in the later decades of life. The sugar content varies from 50 to 80 mg per 100 ml, the precise level being determined by the concentration in the blood; since the CSF sugar generally ranges from 50 to 65 percent of the blood glucose, determination of the latter should always be carried out simultaneously with the lumbar puncture. Tests for syphilis are, of course, negative. In rare instances the chloride content is sought; this ranges normally from 725 to 750 mg per 100 ml. The colloidal gold test, widely regarded as an indirect measure of gamma globulin content, has been largely supplanted by immunoelectrophoresis. Normally, the gamma globulin level is under 12 percent of the total protein content; above 14 percent is clearly abnormal and the range of 12 to 14 percent represents a borderline zone.

Smear and culture of the spinal fluid are indicated in suspected instances of nervous system infection and must be performed before antimicrobial or antibiotic therapy is instituted. Bacteria may be demonstrated by smear in many infections of the meninges, but on occasion are found only with great difficulty; tubercle bacilli are particularly elusive. Viruses are of course not found in this fashion. Parasites, yeasts, and fungi may be found on routine smear rarely, but often require special staining techniques, for example, India ink in instances of torula (cryptococcal) meningitis.

*Abnormalities* of the spinal fluid are found under many circumstances; a search for such variations constitutes an important aspect of the investigation of disease of the nervous system.

### APPEARANCE

The normal CSF is clear and colorless. It may be opalescent or turbid because of accumulation of cells, either red or white. In cases of hemorrhage it is bloody, and the supernatant fluid is generally yellow, or *xanthochromic;* xanthochromia usually results from the breakdown of blood pigments and becomes manifest, at least minimally, within hours of the appearance of blood in the spinal fluid. Xanthochromia may also be noted in instances of subarachnoid block or other conditions characterized by very high protein content. The term *Froin's syndrome* refers to xanthochromic CSF with a high protein content, generally found below the level of a complete subarachnoid block; the xanthochromic CSF coagulates on standing.

## PRESSURE

Disturbances of CSF pressure are found in many conditions. Increased pressure is found in: (1) brain tumor, although not invariably. It is often elevated with posterior fossa tumors, especially those involving the cerebellum, and in many instances of tumor involving the cerebral hemispheres. It is usually normal with tumors in or near the pituitary. (2) Other mass lesions simulating brain tumor, such as epidural or subdural hematoma or brain abscess. (3) Brain edema accompanying or resulting from infection, head injury, cerebral hemorrhage or thrombosis, subarachnoid hemorrhage, and many metabolic encephalopathies. (4) Interference with CSF circulation in obstructive hydrocephalus. (5) Interference with venous outflow, such as thrombosis of the dural venous channels. (6) Pseudotumor cerebri, so-called benign intracranial hypertension.

Decreased pressure (below 100 mm) is found in states of dehydration or in instances in which the spinal fluid column has been shortened as a result of block along the subarachnoid space, as in cases of spinal cord tumor. The spinal fluid pressure may also appear low merely because the needle is not in free communication with the subarachnoid space.

## CELLS

The cell content of the CSF is increased in many conditions. A white cell content of more than six cells is abnormal, while red cells in any amount are of pathologic significance, provided they are not the result of a traumatic puncture. At times, when the CSF contains both white cells and red cells, one must determine whether the leukocytes simply reflect the presence of blood, or whether there is an associated inflammatory response. This dilemma may be resolved simply by bearing in mind that in whole blood there are approximately 700 to 1000 erythrocytes for every leukocyte. This formula can be applied to the WBC/RBC ratio in CSF in any given case to determine the relative importance of the leukocytes therein.

Acute meningeal infections are invariably associated with cell increase; the type and number of cells depends on the cause of the meningitis. Acute *bacterial* infections result in an increase of polymorphonuclear leukocytes in the spinal fluid, whereas *viral* infections are associated with increase in lymphocytes (although polymorphonuclears may appear very early in the course of viral disease, as in the first few hours of infection with poliomyelitis virus). Lymphocytic pleocytosis is not restricted to viral infections of the nervous system. It is found in granulomatous infections, such as neurosyphilis or tuberculous meningitis; in other chronic meningitides, such as cryptococcal meningitis; in invasion of the meninges by neoplastic cells, as in so-called carcinomatosis or lymphomatosis of the meninges, or leukemic meningitis. Lymphocytes also appear in the CSF during recovery from acute bacterial meningitis. Finally, lymphocytes may appear as a nonspecific inflammatory response in the face of tissue necrosis of diverse cause.

## PROTEIN

An *increase* of protein is similarly found under many circumstances. It occurs in both acute and chronic meningitis, in meningeal hemorrhage, in some tumors (particularly those lying close to pial or ependymal surfaces, or in the cerebellopontine angle), in demyelinating disorders, in degenerative disease of various sorts, and in block of the spinal subarachnoid space caused by cord tumor or other obstructing lesions. It may be elevated in diseases of spinal roots or peripheral nerves, as in the Guillain-Barré syndrome of acute "infectious" polyradiculoneuritis (the elevated protein content in the absence of an increase in cells under these circumstances is referred to as *albuminocytologic dissociation*), and is frequently increased in diabetics, even those without neurologic complications. In multiple sclerosis, an increase of the gamma globulin, and particularly of the $\gamma$G fraction, to above 14 percent of the total protein is common and is of particular diagnostic significance when the total protein content falls within the normal range. An oligoclonal electrophoretic pattern is common. An elevated gamma globulin is also typically encountered in subacute sclerosing panencephalitis (SSPE) and in neurosyphilis and occasionally in the Guillain-Barré syndrome or systemic gammopathies such as multiple myeloma. It is apparent, therefore, that an increase in CSF protein may be found in many disorders, but is of specific diagnostic significance in few. Nonetheless, an increased protein content must always be considered abnormal and when found should not be dismissed without an adequate explanation of its occurrence.

A *reduction* in CSF protein is uncommon; it may be found in association with severe liver disease, in which it presumably reflects defective protein synthesis.

## SUGAR

The sugar content of the CSF may be increased or decreased and is dependent ordinarily on blood sugar levels. An *increase* of sugar is of no diagnostic value. *Decreased* sugar content is found in acute bacterial meningitis, in tuberculous meningitis, and in meningeal carcinomatosis or lymphomatosis. In viral meningoencephalitis, on the other hand, the sugar is generally normal; in mumps meningoencephalitis, however, and in herpes simplex encephalitis, the sugar may be reduced. In general, a decreased sugar content is in itself of little diagnostic significance unless accompanied by other abnormalities such as increase of white cells. Again, the necessity for determining the blood sugar simultaneously with the spinal fluid sugar must be emphasized.

## CHLORIDE

Although decreased to some extent with many infections, a serious decrease in CSF chloride was once thought a major if not pathognomonic feature of tuberculous meningitis. In fact, the chloride level in spinal fluid appears to follow the blood level fairly closely, and a reduction is an invariable accompaniment of the hypochloremia attendant upon recurrent vomiting and debilitation. A determination of the spinal fluid chloride is thus of no real diagnostic significance and is only rarely carried out.

## COLLOIDAL GOLD

This test too has largely been discarded, having been replaced by determination of the gamma globulin (see above). Indeed, the colloidal gold test is regarded as an indirect measurement of the level of gamma globulin. For purposes of reference, instances of the "orthodox" patterns of the colloidal gold curve (of Lange) are as follows: (1) first zone (paretic) curve: 5555543210; (2) second zone (tabetic) curve: 1233321000; (3) third zone (meningitic) curve: 0000012310. Numerical values of up to 2 on the usual scale of 0 to 5 cannot be considered abnormal. The most consistent abnormality of the colloidal gold curve is encountered in general paresis; a first zone curve is found in fully 90 percent of untreated cases. Abnormalities are also found in a variety of other circumstances, such as other categories of neurosyphilis, multiple sclerosis, and at times in brain tumor or in tuberculous meningitis.

# ELECTROENCEPHALOGRAPHY

Electroencephalography consists of the amplification, recording, and analysis of the electrical potentials generated by the brain. The electrical activity as recorded from the usual scalp electrodes is not that of the individual neurons but represents, rather, a synthesis of the activity of many neurons, both cortical and, at least indirectly, deep. Sensory stimulation and motor activity alter the ordinary scalp recording relatively little. The basic resting rhythm is, however, affected by opening the eyes and by alteration in attention. When the subject opens his eyes, a prompt decrease in amplitude of the recorded brain waves ensues (the alerting response), with desynchronization of the tracing. The same effect is produced by mental attention, such as computation of a difficult problem.

For proper interpretation the electroencephalogram (EEG) must be used in conjunction with the clinical history and examination, and with other studies. There are few instances in which the EEG has absolute diagnostic value, and evaluation of cerebral disease by means of the EEG alone should be avoided. Even in epilepsy, in which the EEG plays its most significant role, it cannot be considered of unequivocal diagnostic significance; in fact, normal or nondiagnostic EEG records occur in patients with all types of seizures, reflecting the intermittent nature of the disease process. The EEG thus is a supplement to, not a replacement for, careful clinical study.

Electroencephalographic records are obtained over relatively long periods and thus demand a constant yet inexpensive method of recording. Electromagnetic ink writers faithfully reproduce waves varying in frequency from less than 1 in 3 seconds to 30 per second. Amplification is necessary, since the average voltage of the cortical potentials is about 50 to 100 microvolts. Electrodes are generally placed in accordance with the internationally accepted 10–20 system (Fig. 4-1). For special purposes, nasopharyngeal or sphenoidal electrodes are utilized. Tracings are obtained by recording the potential differences from scalp electrodes to ear electrode (monopolar recording) and from scalp electrode to scalp electrode (bipolar recording). Ideally, the patient should be comfortable, quiet, and relaxed, with eyes closed, but not asleep except for specific purposes as noted below. At times, of course, as when portable EEG studies are being carried out in an intensive care unit, such conditions clearly cannot be met.

The most characteristic feature of the normal adult record obtained under standard resting conditions is the 8½ to 12 cycle per second (cps or $H_z$) alpha rhythm (Figs. 4-2 and 4-3). This is usually seen best in the occipital leads, with higher frequency and lower voltage (beta) predominating in the frontal regions and mixtures of alpha, beta, and theta (4-7 cps) in the temporal leads. At birth, frequencies of 1 to 3 cps predominate; active and quiet sleep dominate the tracing in newborns and prematures. With increasing age, the trend is towards faster frequencies, so that by 14 years of age largely adult-type records are obtained, al-

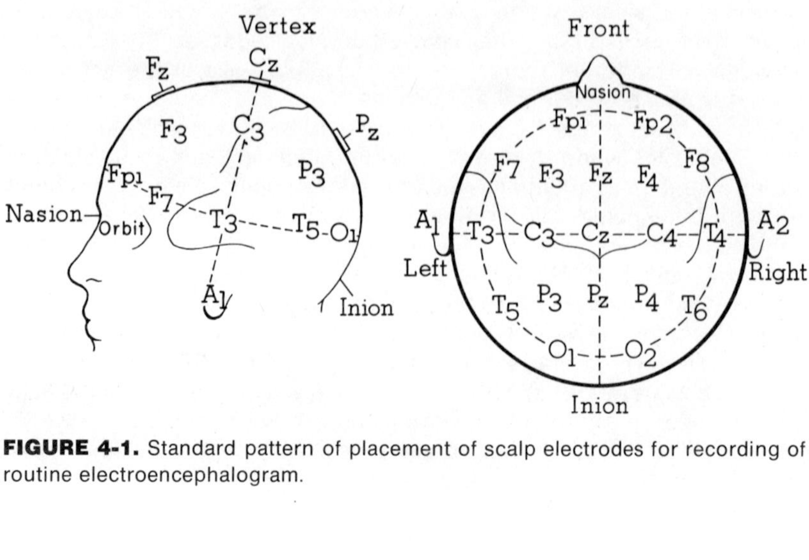


**FIGURE 4-1.** Standard pattern of placement of scalp electrodes for recording of routine electroencephalogram.

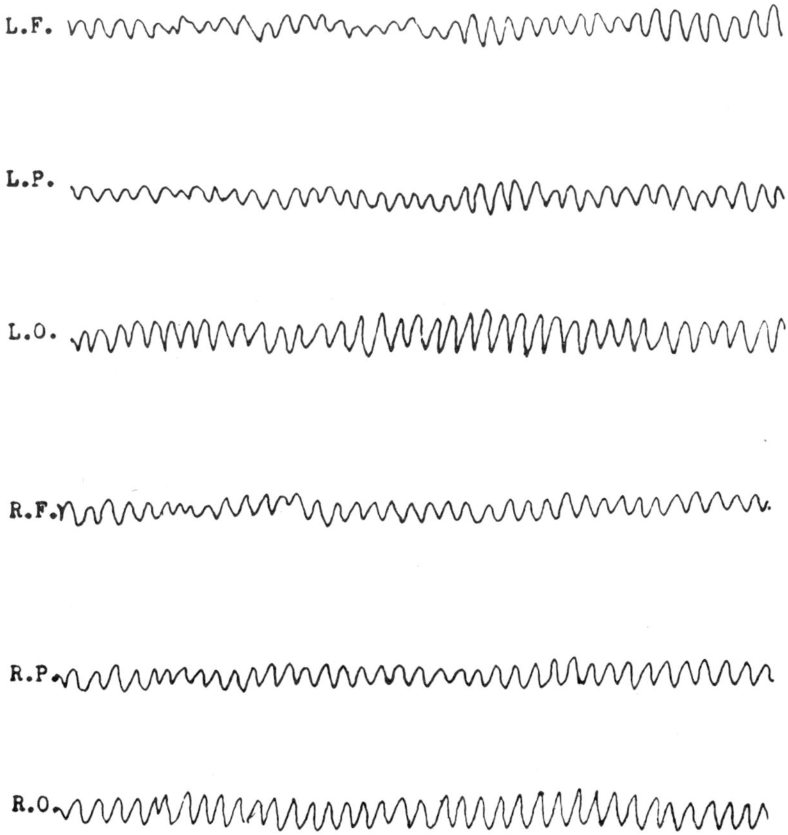


**FIGURE 4-2.** Electroencephalogram, showing normal 8-10/sec. rhythm in frontal, parietal, and occipital areas of the cortex.

though with some persistent childhood features. The frontal and parietal regions are generally the last to evidence adult electrical characteristics; final maturation of the record is evident by 25 years. There is considerable individual variation in the electroencephalographic pattern; a common variant is one of low voltage with rapid frequencies in all leads.

A regular pattern of EEG changes is associated with normal sleep (Fig. 4-4). As the individual falls asleep, the waking EEG is replaced by a stage 1 pattern of low voltage with mixed frequencies. In stage 2, 12 to 14 cps sleep spindles appear, which are accompanied by high voltage complex slow waves called K-complexes, and vertex sharp waves. As the patient descends into deeper sleep (stages 3 and 4), the EEG exhibits increasing high amplitude slow activity, which comes to dominate the tracing in stage 4. REM (rapid eye movement) sleep is characterized electroencephalographically by a return to a stage 1 EEG pattern, with

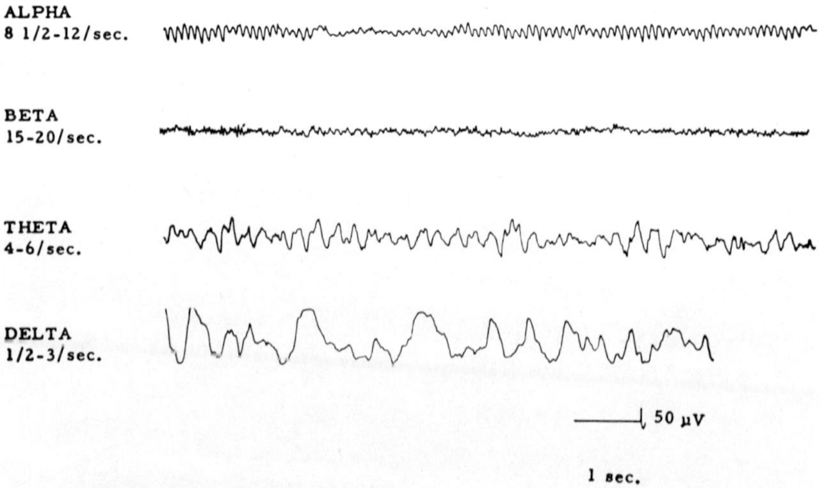


**FIGURE 4-3.** Range of frequencies in the electroencephalogram.

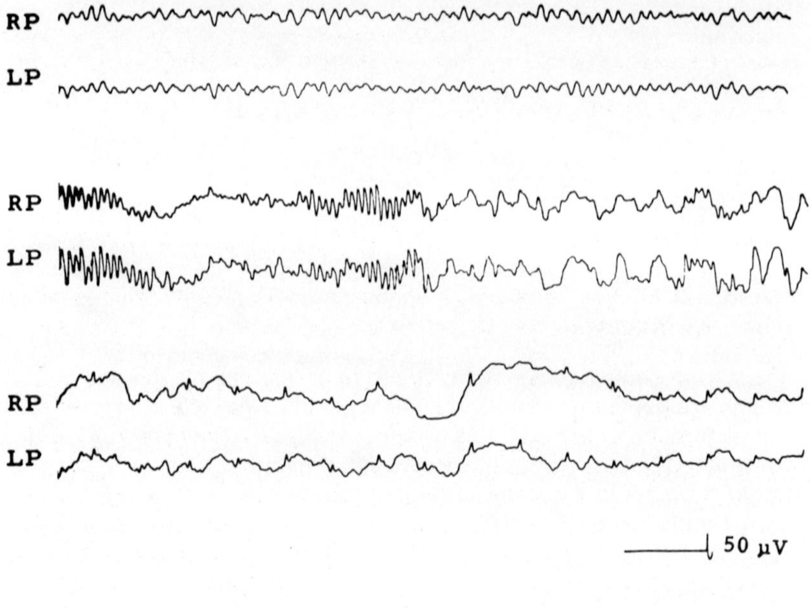


**FIGURE 4-4.** Development of sleep as seen in interrupted records from the right (RP) and left (LP) parietal leads. The irregular mild slowing and low amplitude of sleep onset (Stage 1) give way to 14/sec sleep spindles and so-called K-complexes (Stage 2), which in turn are followed by high voltage slow waves in deep sleep (Stages 3 and 4). In REM (rapid eye movement) sleep, the EEG pattern is similar to that of Stage 1.

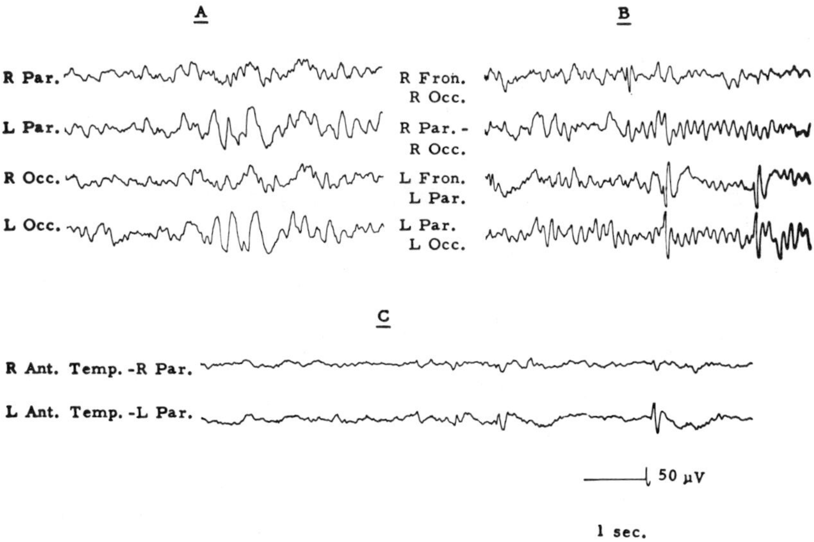


**FIGURE 4-5.** Focal activity in the EEG, arising spontaneously (*A* and *B*) and during sleep activation *(C)*. *A,* High voltage slow waves arise principally from the left hemisphere and are most pronounced in the parietal and occipital leads. *B,* Sharp spike-like waves arise from the left parietal lead. Phase reversal can be identified at the common electrode, a feature of major localizing value. *C,* During sleep temporal lobe discharges may be observed in a patient with psychomotor (complex partial) seizures.

characteristic "saw-tooth" waves that are accompanied by rapid or phasic eye movements, generalized loss of muscle tone, alterations in respiratory and cardiac function, and dreaming. REM sleep recurs on a cyclical basis throughout the period of sleep, alternating with non-REM patterns and increasing in duration as the night's sleep progresses. In the evaluation of sleep disorders, such as narcolepsy, all-night sleep studies (polysonography) and supplemental study of daytime multiple sleep latencies are of major importance.

The electroencephalogram is particularly helpful to the clinician in the diagnosis of epilepsy and the differential diagnosis of seizure disorders, as well as in the localization of lesions of the cerebrum (Fig. 4-5). During epileptic seizures, more or less typical electroencephalographic patterns are encountered (Fig. 4-6). Thus, a generalized tonic-clonic (grand mal) seizure is characterized by fast, high voltage spikes observed in all leads, at times beginning with a focal or lateralizing predominance. In petit mal (absence) attacks, generalized 3 cps spike and wave complexes appear, beginning and ending abruptly with the seizure. In psychomotor seizures (temporal lobe seizures, partial seizures with complex symptomatology), spike discharges in the temporal leads are usual. Nasopharyngeal and/or sphenoidal electrodes are particularly helpful in locat-

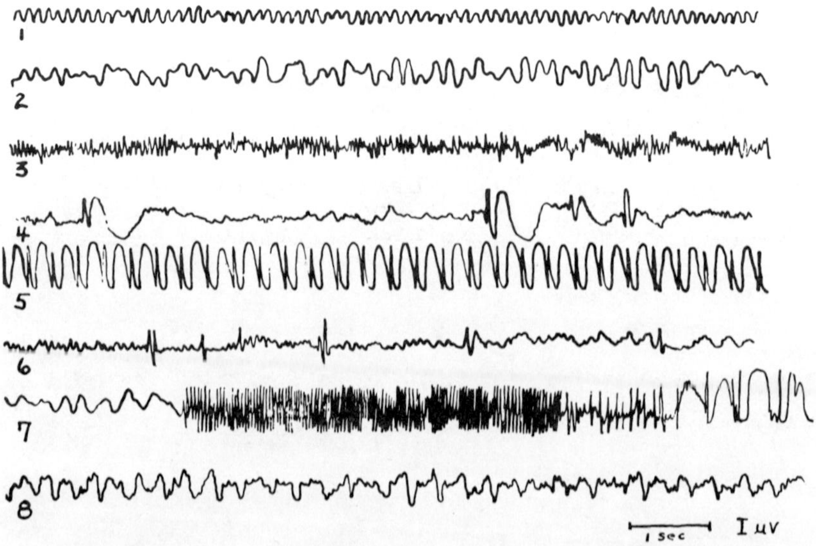


**FIGURE 4-6.** Normal and abnormal cerebral rhythms. 1. Normal alpha rhythm. 2. Slow irregular waves. 3. Fast waves or discharges. 4. Spike and wave, petit mal variant. 5. Spike and wave, petit mal discharge. 6. Spike discharges. 7. Grand mal discharge. 8. Psychomotor discharge at 4-6/sec.

ing discharges from mesial temporal structures. In interseizure records in epileptic patients, isolated spikes or spike-wave complexes may be found; such discharges may also occur in short groups without clinical evidence of a seizure. In patients with petit mal epilepsy, the classical 3 cps spike and wave form may be induced by hyperventilation. In 30 to 50 percent of all epileptic patients, the EEG record between attacks is nonspecific or shows no abnormality. When abnormalities are found, the EEG may contribute to the localization of the epileptogenic focus; thus, localized slowing without spikes may be seen over inactive seizure sites. In some patients, extended study that utilizes simultaneous EEG and video recording is of major diagnostic assistance.

Various methods of inducing electroencephalographic abnormalities are utilized. Hyperventilation has long been recognized as of value in eliciting typical petit mal discharges. Recording during drowsiness and sleep may bring out abnormal discharges in all types of epilepsy, particularly in temporal lobe (partial complex) seizures. Photic stimulation may similarly activate the EEG and at times induce a frank seizure. Carefully controlled intravenous injection of Metrazol has been found efficacious in demonstrating epileptogenic foci, but is only rarely used.

Gross lesions of the cerebral hemispheres that lie within the range of the scalp electrodes may be localized by means of electroencephalography. For example, delta activity ($1/2$ to 3 cps waves of high voltage) may be found in relation to the electrode(s) over infarction, hemorrhage, tumor, or abscess. The closer the lesion to the surface of the hemisphere, the more clear-cut and reliable is the localization; deep-seated cerebral and midline lesions are localized much more poorly than those more superficially placed. When the lesion is in the posterior fossa, little assistance is derived from the EEG in terms of localization.

In addition, the EEG is often helpful in a variety of other circumstances, such as in instances of head injury or of metabolic encephalopathies (demonstrating, for example, the triphasic waves most typical of hepatic coma), and may be very useful in assessing the depth of coma. Generalized periodic discharges separated by periods of electrical silence appear in a variety of circumstances, as in subacute sclerosing panencephalitis (SSPE), in the neuronal lipidoses, in Jakob-Creutzfeldt disease, and in other diffuse gray matter disorders. Under some circumstances, as with subdural hematoma or in the face of extensive cerebral infarction, a reduction of electrical activity is observed, and a very low voltage high frequency record is often described in Huntington's disease. Finally, as previously noted, the importance of a persistent isoelectric tracing as confirmatory evidence of brain death cannot be overestimated, particularly as regards selection of patients as donors for organ transplant.

The results of electroencephalographic study in psychiatric disorders are inconclusive. Thus, while there are more frequent although nonspecific EEG abnormalities in the major psychoses, it is impossible to establish the presence of a psychosis, much less its type, by the record of an individual patient. As would be anticipated, abnormalities of the EEG are more common in psychoses associated with organic brain disease. Attempts at correlating EEG patterns with intelligence level in retarded individuals have also been unsuccessful. The greater incidence of abnormalities in those with very low intelligence is more likely correlated with the underlying cerebral disease than with the intelligence level *per se*. A high incidence of nonspecific abnormalities has also been demonstrated in children with behavioral problems.

## Evoked Responses

Determination of evoked responses (event-related brain potentials) has become increasingly useful in neurologic diagnosis. In brief, an evoked response is by definition the transient brain potential, expressed as a sudden change in the brain waves, that results from the application of a brief external stimulus. By applying contemporary computer technology, utilizing response-averaging techniques with a large number of stimuli, it is possible to extract the signal (i.e., the stimulus-evoked activity) from the background electroencephalographic "noise"; both the amplitude and the latency of such a stimulus-evoked response can be measured. This technique provides an objective measurement of the functional status of at least certain afferent sensory pathways. Three forms of evoked response determinations are presently suitable for clinical application:

1. Determination of the *visual evoked responses* utilizes as a stimulus either a bright flash or, more reliably, pattern (checkerboard) reversal. Responses vary, depending upon whether the lesion involves the retina, the optic nerve, or the postchiasmatic visual conducting system. A delay in latency is typical of optic nerve disease and is found most frequently in patients with multiple sclerosis, even in the absence of a history of visual impairment. This therefore comprises a useful ancillary laboratory procedure in the diagnosis of demyelinating disease. Other disorders such as pernicious anemia produce similar results. The technique also permits monitoring of optic nerve or chiasmatic compression by tumor, such as a pituitary adenoma, and provides an objective measurement of the efficacy of treatment in such cases.

2. *Auditory evoked potentials* are click-induced and provide useful information in disorders of the cochlea, of the auditory nerve, and of the central (particularly brainstem) connections. This procedure may be of great assistance in assessing deafness in infants, the mentally retarded, autistic children, or in others in whom audiometry is not feasible or reliable. Variations in the central conduction time may be noted in patients with lesions such as multiple sclerosis or brainstem tumor.

3. *Somatosensory evoked responses* are responses to electrical or, less commonly, tactile stimulation at the periphery. Significant delays are found in both peripheral and central lesions. Such responses may be of assistance in distinguishing between organic and hysterical sensory loss.

## ELECTROMYOGRAPHY

Electromyography consists essentially of the observation and recording of electrical potentials derived from or arising within individual muscle fibers; such potentials are initially detected by needle electrodes, amplified electronically, and ultimately displayed on an oscilloscope and loudspeaker. Various photographic and electronic techniques permit storage of permanent records. In the normal and in a number of disease states a variety of individually identifiable potentials can be recognized, whose principle characteristics may be summarized as follows:

When the needle electrode is originally placed within the muscle, *insertional activity* appears, which comprises potentials evoked by injury to the muscle fiber; at times, nerve potentials and miniature end-plate potentials (sometimes referred to as end-plate noise) appear at this time as well. When insertional activity has subsided, and the needle movement has ceased, and the muscle remains at repose, spontaneously arising potentials may appear in certain pathologic states. These include: (1) *Positive sharp waves,* nonpropagated potentials that vary in amplitude from 50 to 1000 microvolts with a duration of 10 milliseconds or more. Needle movement may stimulate the appearance of these potentials. Positive sharp waves are not found in the normal; their appearance is most suggestive of denervation. (2) *Fibrillation potentials,* which consist of short duration biphasic or triphasic waves with irregular firing at rates of 2 to 20 per second and varying in amplitude from 20 to 300 microvolts. These are commonly, although not invariably, associated with denervation or with inflammatory muscle diseases or other subacute myopathies. (3) *Fasciculation potentials,* large and at times rhythmic potentials of varying form that represent the summation of a number of individual motor unit potentials, those potentials generated by the spontaneous firing of a single motor unit or a group of several units. Characteristically encountered in motor system disease and in other conditions characterized by damaged anterior horn cells or motor nerve roots, fasciculation potentials may also be seen in hyperthyroidism, uremia, the syndrome of benign myokymia, and, on occasion, in normal individuals. (4) *Myotonic discharges,* high frequency discharges that occur in trains of potentials, varying in amplitude, and appearing particularly with electrode movement. Rates of up to 150 per second may be found. Typically there is a rapid rise and a nearly as rapid fall in frequency; over the loudspeaker, these potential sequences cause a rising and falling sound reminiscent of that of a dive bomber.

After a careful search has been made for such spontaneous electrical activity, volitional movements are undertaken to elicit true action potentials. Isolated *action potentials* are best studied with minimal voluntary contraction; they appear as diphasic or triphasic waves of 4 to 10 millisecond duration and vary in amplitude from 300 microvolts to 2 millivolts. With increasing voluntary activity, individual action potentials build up, ultimately with maximal effort fusing in a so-called *interference pattern.*

Response of the pattern of action potentials to *repetitive stimulation* of the muscle is also investigated. Deviations from normal are encountered, for example, in myasthenia gravis, in which decay in amplitude of successive potentials is seen, and in the Lambert-Eaton syndrome, the "myasthenic" syndrome of carcinoma of the lung, in which the opposite pertains, at least with rapid stimulation.

It must be emphasized that no pattern of muscle action potential is necessary for, or pathognomonic of, any particular disease. *Myopathic* illnesses generally do, however, tend to share certain electromyographic features, although some variability may be found. Insertional activity is commonly normal or nearly so. However, in rapidly evolving disorders such as polymyositis there may be considerable increase in insertional activity, whereas when there has been extensive replacement of muscle by fat or connective tissue, as in the late stages of dystrophy, insertional activity may be severely reduced or absent. During complete relaxation no electrical activity can be recorded in the majority of myopathies. In myotonic dystrophy, however, and in the other myotonic syndromes, post-contraction fibrillation activity is found, which consists of brief showers of small-amplitude very rapid diphasic or triphasic spike potentials presumably representing abnormally persistent activity of individual muscle fibers. Additionally, as noted above, myotonic states are characterized by the presence of high frequency discharges elicited by movement of the electrode, the so-called myotonic discharges. (These features, it should be added, permit identification of myopathies exhibiting myotonia as distinct from other disorders of muscle.) With voluntary contraction, the expected build-up of action potentials with development of an interference pattern that results from the fusion of individual potentials appears and is normal in most myopathies. Characteristically, one encounters rapid and low amplitude potentials. Polyphasic potentials (so-called *disintegrated* or *myopathic potentials),* absent in the normal, are common with myopathy and are of major diagnostic importance. In some myopathies, particularly polymyositis and other subacute disorders, fibrillation potentials may also appear.

In *denervated muscle,* electrical changes are observed that differ markedly from those of myopathy. At rest, spontaneous fibrillation potentials are common, and these small rapid potentials may be so prominent as to replace normal insertional activity. It should be emphasized that the fibrillation potentials do not appear until from 10 to 25 days following axonal interruption. Fasciculation potentials may be seen; as already noted, these are most striking in individuals with disease of the anterior horn cells. Large-amplitude slow positive potentials called positive sharp waves are also characteristically found in instances of denervation. With voluntary contraction, a defective interference pattern is seen, which reflects reduction in the number of available motor units. Polyphasic potentials may also occur, but tend to be only a minor component of the electromyographic constellation of denervation. Electromyographic studies in denervation thus yield substantially different results from those in myopathic disease, and it is in distinguishing the two that such electrophysiologic techniques achieve their most widespread application.

Among other available electrodiagnostic studies, determination of *nerve conduction velocity* is perhaps the most valuable. Techniques are available to assess conduction in both motor and sensory nerves. Conduction rates vary from individual to individual, and from nerve to nerve. In the very young, conduction of the nerve impulse is much slower than in the adult; adult velocities are usually found by the age of 5 years. In the adult, a lower limit of normal for the median or ulnar nerve is 49 meters per second, whereas in the peroneal or tibial nerves the lower limit is 35 meters per second. Recorded velocities are influenced by the temperature of the limbs, and this should be carefully controlled for accurate evaluation. Nerve conduction studies find broadest application in the evaluation of disorders of the peripheral nervous system, but may prove of some limited value in diseases of the spinal roots and of the spinal cord itself. In instances of peripheral neuropathy, a marked slowing in conduction velocity, in the range of 12 to 18 meters per second or less, suggests a demyelinating (segmental, Gombault) type of neuropathy as pertains, for example, in the Guillain-Barré syndrome or in Charcot-Marie-Tooth disease (peroneal muscular atrophy). In contrast, normal or only mildly reduced velocities, for example, in the range of 30 to 40 meters per second, are encountered with so-called axonal (Wallerian) neuropathies, which are exemplified by the polyneuropathies of nutritional depletion, uremia, and diabetes, at least in its early stages.

## BRAIN SCANNING

Radioisotope (scintillation) scanning provides a safe screening procedure in the diagnosis of intracranial lesions and is commonly utilized before

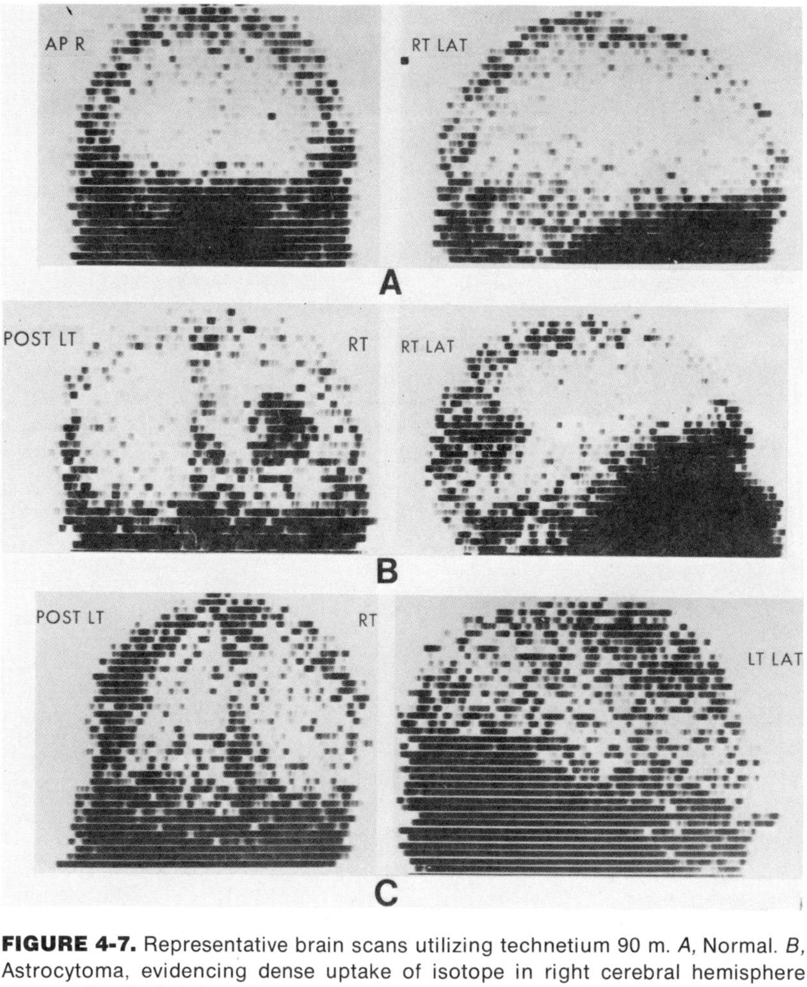


**FIGURE 4-7.** Representative brain scans utilizing technetium 90 m. *A,* Normal. *B,* Astrocytoma, evidencing dense uptake of isotope in right cerebral hemisphere posteriorly. *C,* Subdural hematoma, with prominent peripheral concentration of isotope overlying the left hemisphere. (Courtesy of Dr. Millard Croll)

resorting to contrast studies. A variety of isotopes has been employed for this type of study, originally $^{131}$I-labeled diiodofluorescein and $^{131}$I-labeled serum albumin, more recently $^{203}$Hg-labeled chlormerodrin and $^{99m}$technetium. Scanning techniques delineate abnormal areas of isotope concentration and are most useful with supratentorial lesions. Neoplasms, infarctions, vascular malformations and both intra- and extracerebral hematomas may be demonstrated. Lacerations and hematomas of the scalp may also concentrate the isotope, which leads to occasional errors in interpretation. Because of overlying extracranial muscle masses, which

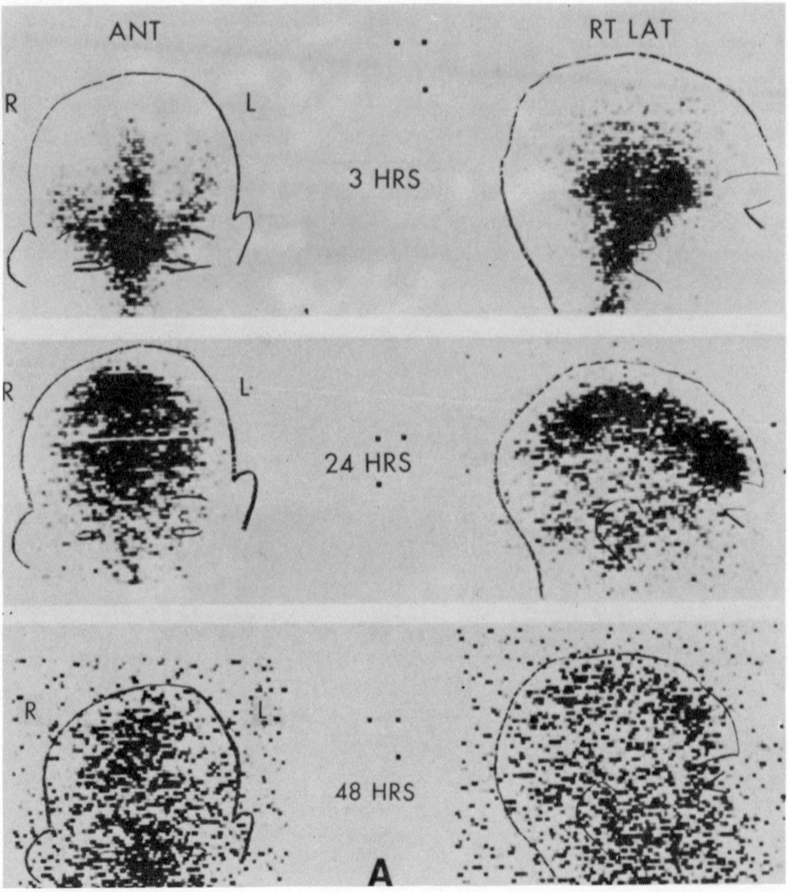


**FIGURE 4-8.** Isotope cisternography. *A,* Normal series at 3, 24, and 48 hours after introduction of the isotope into the lumbar subarachnoid space. Isotope is present in the basal cisterns and to some extent the ventricles at 3 hours, but has largely migrated to the convexity of the hemispheres by 24 hours. Only a small amount of isotope is present at 48 hours.

may mask underlying concentrations of the isotope, scans are much less informative when dealing with lesions at the base of the skull and in the posterior fossa. With the advent of computerized tomography, isotopic scanning has lost considerable ground as a diagnostic tool. It remains valuable, however, in the diagnosis of certain tumors, in particular metastatic carcinoma, and in the definition of other lesions such as subdural hematomas, which may be "isodense" with computerized tomographic techniques and thus difficult or impossible to visualize (Fig. 4-7).

Another isotopic scanning procedure of value is *isotope cistern-*

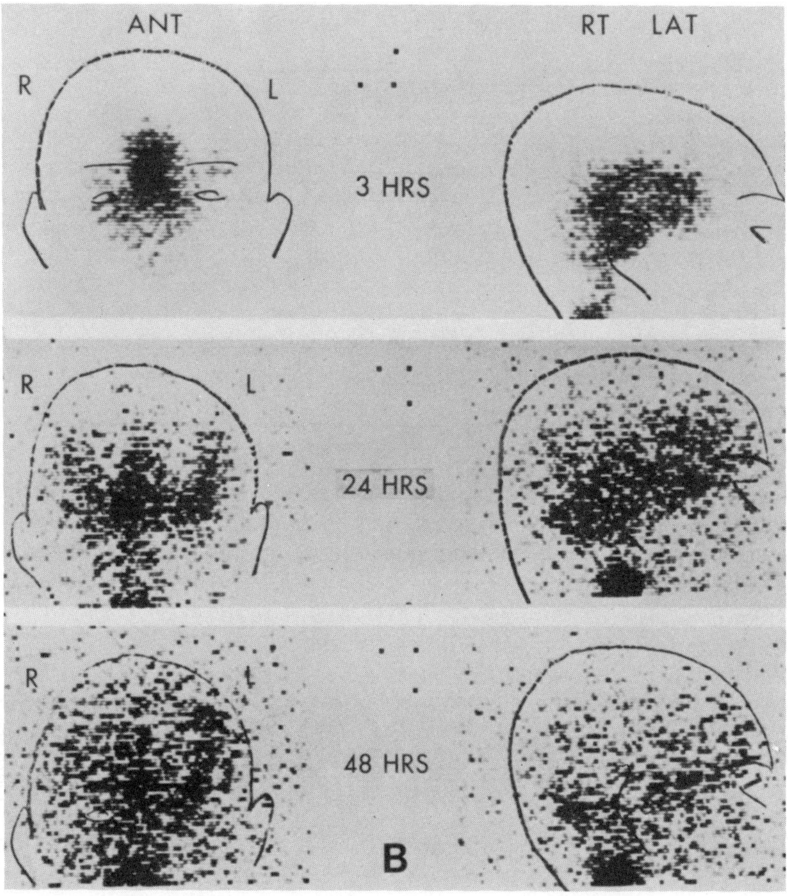


**FIGURE 4-8** *(continued). B,* Occult (normal pressure) hydrocephalus. Marked delay in migration of the isotope is observed. A strong concentration is still evident within the basal cisterns and ventricles at 24 hours, with virtually none over the convexities. Even at 48 hours a substantial amount of isotope remains concentrated within the ventricles. (Courtesy of Dr. Millard Croll)

*ography,* especially in instances of occult (normal pressure) hydrocephalus and other conditions in which a dynamic visualization of the cerebrospinal fluid pathways may be informative. The isotope, generally Indium ($^{111}$In-DTPA) is injected into the lumbar subarachnoid space. With serial scans, the migration of the isotope is monitored as it enters the subarachnoid cisterns at the base of the brain, passes over the convexities of the hemispheres, and finally enters the superior sagittal sinus. In cases of obstruction of flow over the convexities, as in instances of incisural block, the isotope lingers for protracted periods within the basal cisterns, concentrates in large quantities within the ventricles, and traverses the cerebral subarachnoid pathways only with considerable delay (Fig. 4-8).

## ECHOENCEPHALOGRAPHY

Echoencephalography is sometimes used as part of a preliminary screening in the search for intracranial disease. Utilizing ultrasonic techniques for the recording of echoes derived from deep structures within the cranial cavity, this procedure is most valuable in identifying the midline (Fig. 4-9) and, thus, in documenting a shift of the cranial contents from one side to the other in expanding lesions such as subdural hematomas. The contour of the ventricular system and even the thickness of intracranial hematomas can sometimes be demonstrated by experienced investigators utilizing this technique.

## MYELOGRAPHY

Pantopaque, metrizamide (Amipaque), or some other hyperbaric radiopaque substance may be injected into the subarachnoid space to create a contrast medium against which defects within the spinal canal may be visualized. The dye is introduced generally by lumbar puncture, occasionally via the cisternal route. The volume of contrast material utilized varies; for lumbar myelography, a relatively small amount of dye is re-

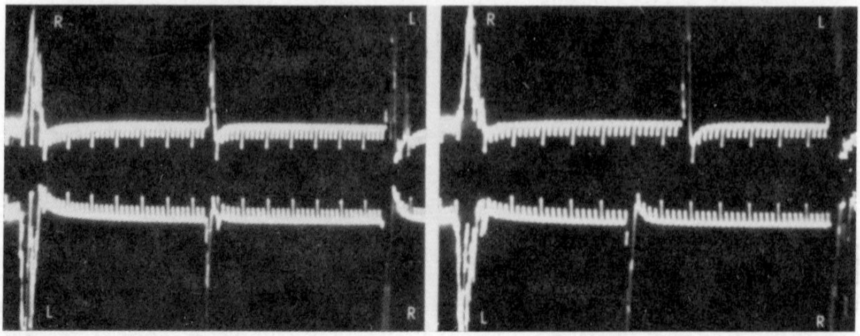


**FIGURE 4-9.** Echoencephalogram. Left: Normal tracing. Right: Deviation of midline (falx) from right to left. (Courtesy of Dr. Carlos F. Gonzalez)

quired, whereas for thoracic and cervical studies substantially more is necessary. Following radiographic study, agents such as Pantopaque are usually removed as completely as possible; when a complete or nearly complete spinal block has been demonstrated, however, removal of the oil with any degree of suction may be dangerous and should be avoided. Metrizamide, on the other hand, appears to be completely resorbed from the subarachnoid space within a relatively short period of time and thus does not require mechanical removal.

The contrast media employed in myelography are not biologically inert, and their use is not free of hazard. Meningeal irritation with frank sterile meningitis is common after use of such agents. Local root irritation is frequent, and radicular pain may linger for some time. Rarely, progressive adhesive arachnoiditis characterized by root pain, weakness, sensory loss, and sphincter disorder appears as a delayed complication of the procedure. In an effort to avoid such side effects, air myelography has been utilized, but poses formidable technical problems. Metrizamide is

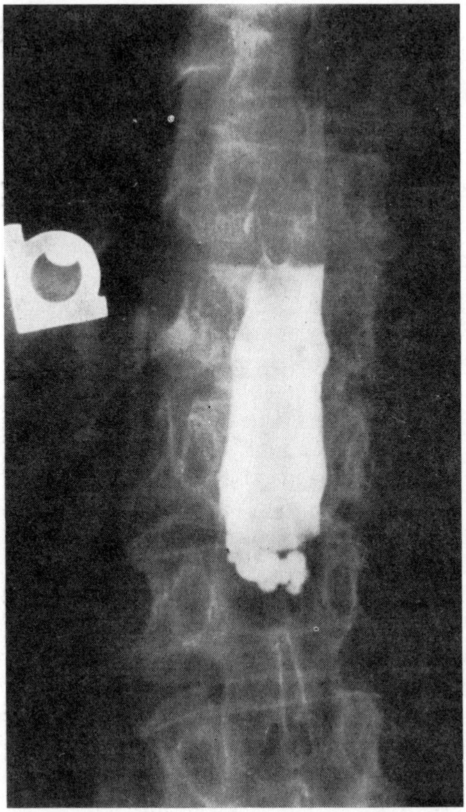

**FIGURE 4-10.** Pantopaque myelogram revealing complete block due to extramedullary meningioma.

in general a much less irritating contrast medium. Unfortunately, when metrizamide enters the cranial vault it may on rare occasions precipitate a generalized seizure, especially in those with a known epileptic potential. Since intracranial movement of the dye in relatively high concentrations often occurs in cervical myelography, its use here is discouraged; when this is necessary, however, the patient should be prepared with an anticonvulsant such as phenobarbital.

In cases of complete block of the subarachnoid pathways, arrest of the contrast medium is seen (Fig. 4-10). In incomplete block some oil escapes around the obstruction, although its movement may be slow. The precise configuration of the radiographic deficit is often of material assistance in determining whether the offending lesion is intramedullary or extramedullary, and, if the latter, subdural or epidural. On occasion, particularly when a vascular malformation of the spinal cord is suspected, the lesion may be missed entirely unless the lumbar needle is removed, the patient turned over, and fluoroscopic examination repeated with the patient lying on his back.

Myelography may also be utilized in the diagnosis of tumors of the posterior fossa, especially acoustic neuromas, in those cases in which other radiographic procedures have failed to document the presence of a neoplasm suspected on clinical and otologic grounds. The opaque oil is maneuvered into the cerebellopontine angle and directly into the acoustic canal for this purpose. Intracanalicular acoustic tumors less than 1 cm in diameter can be demonstrated in this fashion.

## PNEUMOENCEPHALOGRAPHY

Once the most common contrast neuroradiographic procedure, pneumoencephalography has been almost entirely discarded since the advent of computerized tomography. A painful and at times incapacitating procedure, it nonetheless remains a useful investigation in certain selected cases and requires brief comment. The pneumoencephalogram, or air study (Figs. 4-11 and 4-12), has in general been of value in the investigation of atrophic and degenerative disorders of the nervous system, and of hydrocephalus; it has proven of substantial assistance in the diagnosis of suprasellar and posterior fossa lesions as well. Pneumoencephalography is contraindicated in the face of increased intracranial pressure; when necessary, air may be introduced directly into the ventricles from above through burr holes, a method referred to as *ventriculography.* A radiopaque agent, such as Pantopaque or metrizamide, may also be introduced into the lateral ventricle to produce positive contrast ventriculography, at times of benefit when precise delineation of the aqueduct of Sylvius, fourth ventricle, and lateral recesses is required.

The well-recognized patterns of abnormality encountered with the pneumoencephalogram are as follows:

1. In instances of a mass lesion, distortion, obliteration, or displacement of the ventricles is the cardinal abnormality, associated at times with

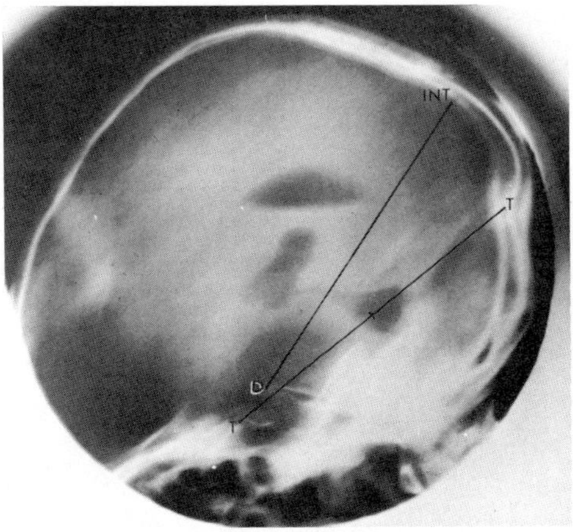


**FIGURE 4-11.** Methods of determining displacement of the aqueduct and fourth ventricle with pneumoencephalography. The line T-T, sometimes called Twining's line, is drawn from the tuberculum sella to the torcular Herophili; its midpoint normally falls within the fourth ventricle, usually close to the floor. The line D-INT originates on the dorsum sella and is projected through the site of junction of aqueduct and fourth ventricle to the inner table of the skull. The aqueduct ordinarily lies where the anterior and middle thirds of this line meet. (Courtesy of Dr. Carlos F. Gonzalez)

more remote alterations such as internal hydrocephalus. Changes in the cisterns may on occasion be found, for example, obliteration of the prepontine cistern in instances of pontine glioma, or alterations of the chiasmatic cistern with suprasellar lesions.

2. Conditions characterized by parenchymatous atrophy such as Alzheimer's disease are recognized by symmetrical enlargement of the ventricular system along with cerebral convolutional atrophy. When such ventricular enlargement develops as a result of loss of nervous tissue, the term *hydrocephalus ex vacuo* is sometimes applied. Focal cerebral atrophy may be encountered, as with a post-traumatic meningocerebral cicatrix, and localized ventricular enlargement may be found under such circumstances; at times, the entire ventricular system is distorted and shifted toward the lesion, as a so-called *atrophic shift.* A frank cyst in communication with the ventricle may appear, termed a *porencephalic cyst.*

3. Arachnoiditis, particularly when it involves the region of the optic chiasm, may also be diagnosed with an air study and is evidenced by failure of filling of the chiasmatic and prechiasmatic cisterns. Arachnoidal abnormalities elsewhere are far more difficult to define.

4. In hydrocephalus, the utility of pneumoencephalography is self-evident, by virtue of the ability of the procedure to outline the ventricles with great precision; the therapeutic importance of identification of the exact site of obstruction of flow of spinal fluid cannot be overestimated.

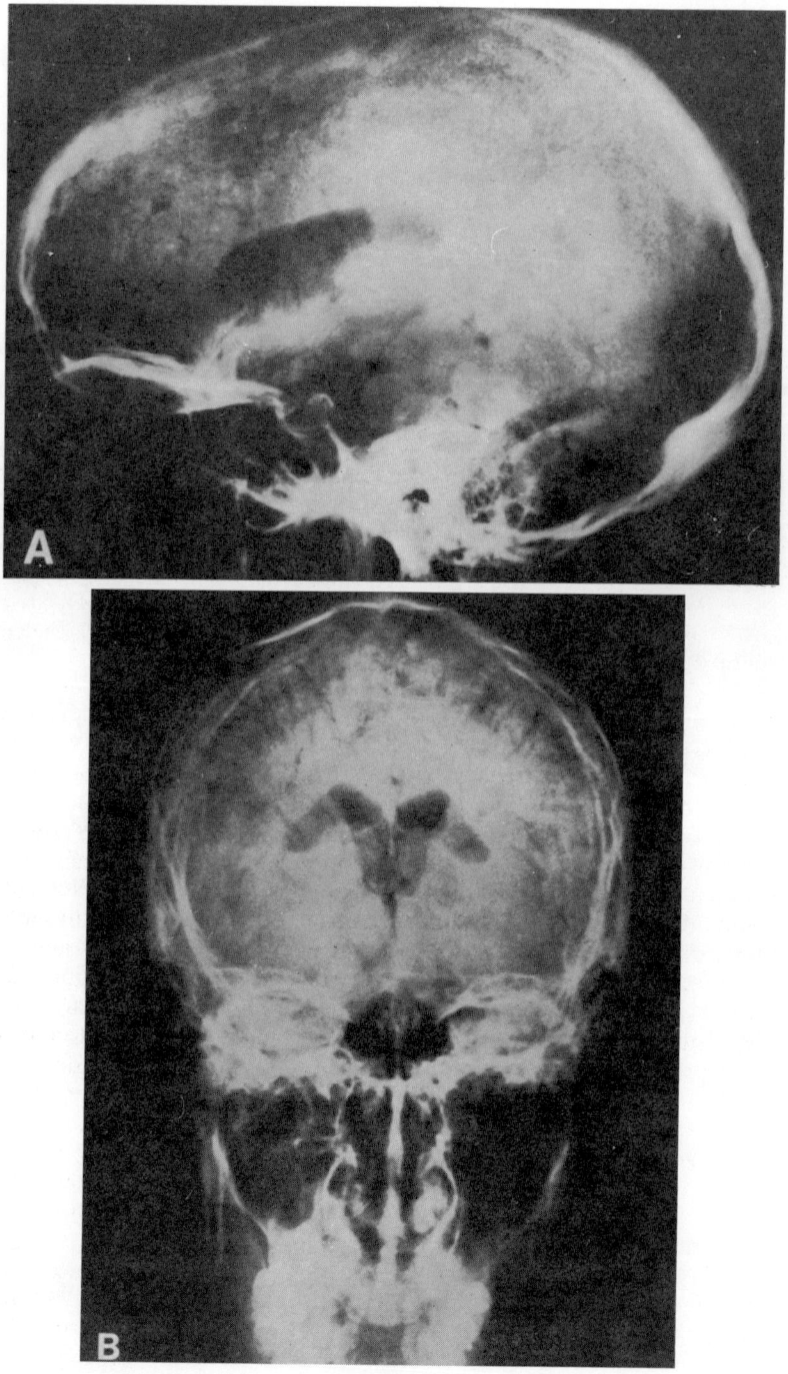
A
B

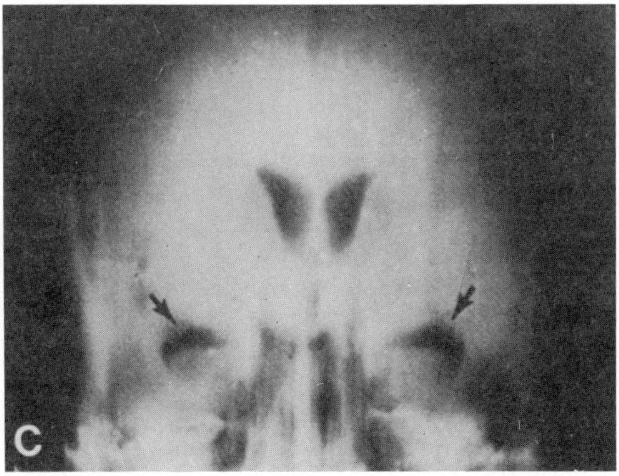

**FIGURE 4-12.** Normal pneumoencephalograms. *A,* Lateral projection in brow-up position. The frontal horns and bodies of the lateral ventricles are well visualized; the occipital horns are not filled with air in this position. The foramen of Monro is clearly seen, and there is a small amount of air in the third ventricle. The pontine, interpeduncular, and chiasmatic cisterns are readily identified at the base. *B,* Anteroposterior projection through the bodies of the lateral ventricles. The third ventricle is seen as a slit in the midline. The origin of the temporal horns is readily identified. *C,* Tomogram in the anteroposterior plane, demonstrating air in the lateral and third ventricles as well as in the temporal horns *(arrows).*

## ARTERIOGRAPHY

Cerebral arteriography (angiography) is ordinarily performed via a femoral catheter with selective arterial injection. It plays an important role in the evaluation of patients with both intracranial and extracranial vascular disease, and, to a lesser extent, with intracranial mass lesions, especially when supratentorial. Assessment of the arterial, capillary, and venous phases of the circulation is permitted (Figs. 4-13 and 4-14), and a rough estimate of circulation time may be made. The dural venous sinuses are also visualized; in some circumstances, direct injection of the superior sagittal sinus itself is warranted (sinogram). In the final analysis, the use of angiography can best be determined by correlating the results of clinical evaluation of the patient with the results of noninvasive testing, including, most importantly, computerized tomography. Angiography, it should be emphasized, does carry certain risks, such as idiosyncratic response to the iodinated dye or dislodgement of an atheromatous plaque by the femoral catheter. The morbidity rate is, however, low (less than 1% in experienced hands).

Alterations visualized with the arteriogram may be considered in three major categories:

1. *Structural abnormalities of vessels.* Changes in the structure of the vessel walls themselves, and in the lumen, are both identifiable. Vas-

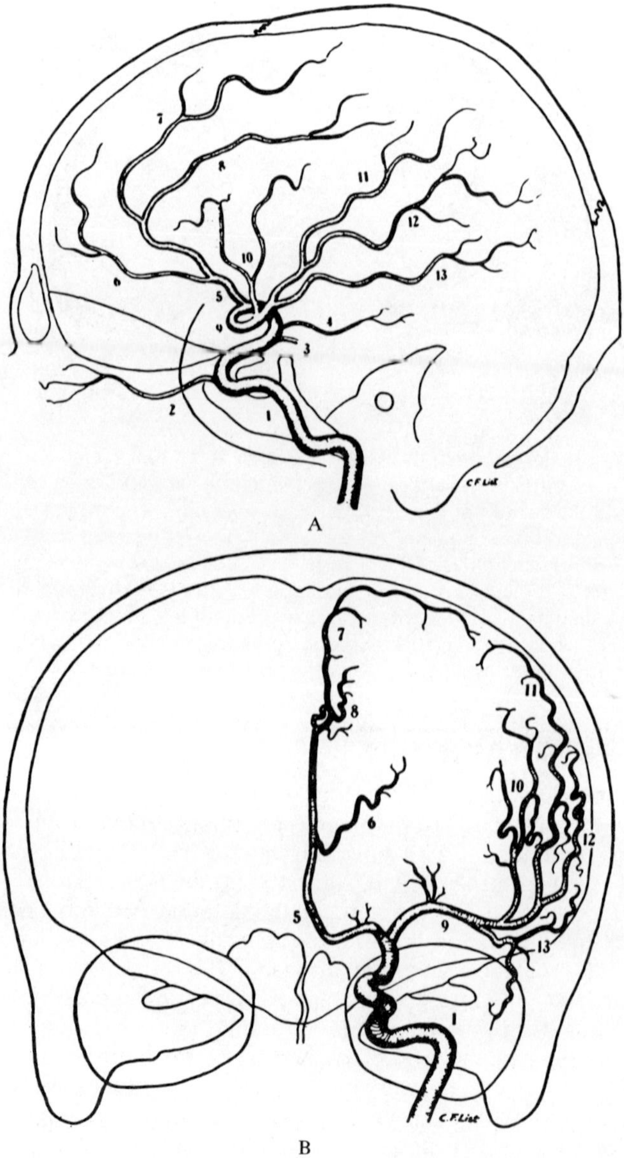


**FIGURE 4-13.** Schematic drawings of normal arteriograms and venogram. *A,* Carotid arteriogram, lateral projection. *B,* Carotid arteriogram, anteroposterior projection. 1. Internal carotid artery. 2. Ophthalmic artery. 3. Posterior communicating artery. 4. Anterior choroidal artery. 5. Anterior cerebral artery. 6. Frontopolar artery. 7. Callosomarginal artery. 8. Pericallosal artery. 9. Middle cerebral artery. 10. Ascending frontoparietal artery. 11. Posterior parietal artery. 12. Angular artery. 13. Posterior temporal artery.

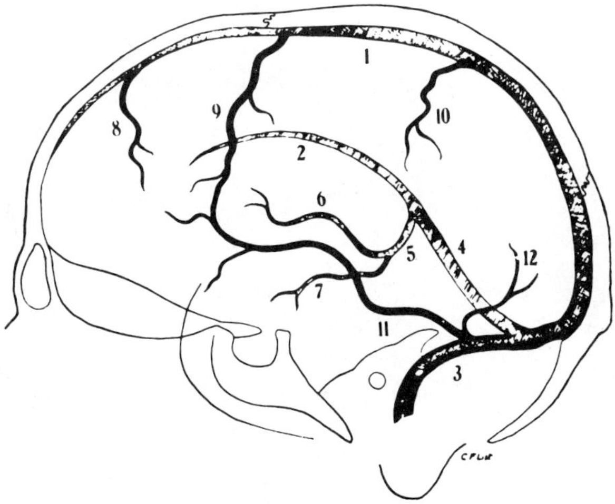


C

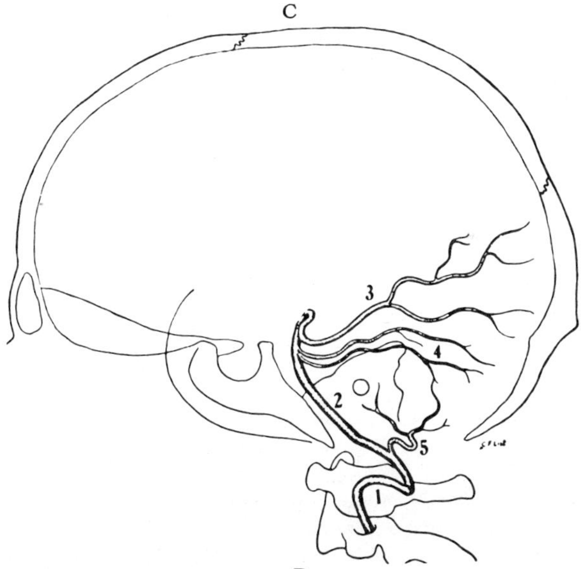


D

**FIGURE 4-13** *(continued). C,* Normal venogram, lateral projection, obtained by carotid injection. Superficial veins are shaded more darkly than sinuses and deep veins. 1. Superior sagittal sinus. 2. Inferior sagittal sinus. 3. Transverse sinus. 4. Straight sinus. 5. Great cerebral vein of Galen. 6. Internal cerebral vein. 7. Basal vein of Rosenthal. 8. Frontal ascending vein. 9. Rolandic vein of Trolard. 10. Parietal ascending vein. 11. Communicating temporal vein of Labbé. 12. Descending temporo-occipital vein. *D,* Normal vertebral arteriogram, lateral projection. 1. Vertebral artery. 2. Basilar artery. 3. Posterior cerebral artery. 4. Superior cerebellar artery. 5. Posterior inferior cerebellar artery. (From List, D. F., Burge, C. H., and Hodges, F. J.: *Intracranial Angiography.* Radiology 45:1, 1945.)

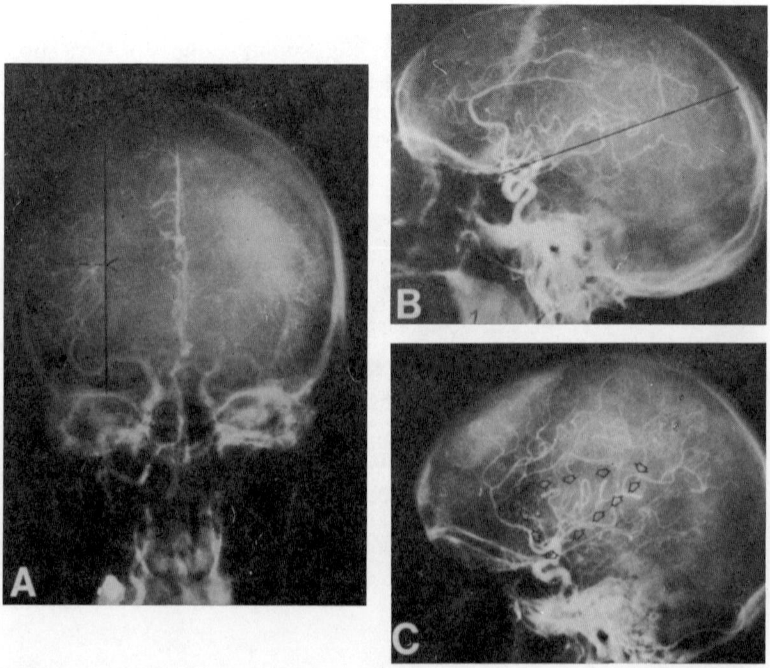


**FIGURE 4-14.** Pertinent landmarks identifiable with the carotid angiogram that are of use in determining the direction and degree of shift of the vascular structures as a result of intracranial disease. *A,* The sylvian point (*arrow*), which represents the mesial curving of the last major sylvian branch of the middle cerebral artery and, thus, the posterior extent of the sylvian fissure. As found in the anteroposterior plane, it lies close to the midpoint of a line connecting the upper margin of the petrous pyramid, or of the roof of the orbit, to a horizontal line drawn tangential to the inner table of the vertex. It is usually 3.0 to 4.3 cm from the inner table of the skull laterally. *B,* The clinoparietal line. Drawn between the anterior clinoid and a point on the calvarium 9.0 cm above the inion, this line roughly parallels the course of the middle cerebral artery; in the adult the artery falls 0.5 cm, or less, above or below. *C,* The sylvian triangle. The components of this complex structure are as follows: The *top* of the triangle follows the tops of the insular loops, that is, the loops of the insular (sylvian) branches of the middle cerebral artery; the *apex,* or posteriormost point, of the triangle is the sylvian point; the *base* comprises a line drawn from the sylvian point to the base of the first ascending insular branch of the middle cerebral artery; the remaining *side* is equivalent to the anterior insular line, running from the origin of the first ascending insular branch to the most anterosuperior insular loop. (Courtesy of Dr. Carlos F. Gonzalez)

cular malformations and aneurysms are obvious instances. Stenotic or thrombosed vessels may be identified, and the characteristics and extent of atherosclerotic plaques defined. In some circumstances, as with subarachnoid hemorrhage caused by rupture of an aneurysm, vascular spasm may be encountered, and segmental zones of narrowing may be seen in instances of cerebral arteritis; in contrast, in other settings widely dilated (ectatic) vessels are sometimes found. Finally, collections of abnormal vessels, often exhibiting unusual patterns of arteriovenous shunting, may be demonstrated within certain neoplasms, in particular gliomas, meningiomas, and metastatic carcinomas, and are responsible for the so-called *tumor blush* or *stain.*

2. *Alterations in position of vessels.* Mass lesions of all sorts produce vascular displacement. Such displacement may be local and result in more or less complete and direct delineation of the mass, or distant and indirect; examples of the latter include shift of the anterior cerebral artery with anteriorly placed mass lesions or of the internal cerebral vein with lesions more posteriorly placed. At times such a shift of vessels is associated with a stain or blush (see above); in other instances, as with subdural or intracerebral hematoma, or brain abscess, only the change in position of the vessels is visualized, the lesion itself being represented by an avascular area. In cases of increased intracranial pressure with internal hydrocephalus, the vessels may be observed to be attenuated and stretched over the dilated ventricles.

3. *Alterations in flow patterns.* Changes in the circulatory pattern may be evident as an expression of abnormal vascular shunts, as with arteriovenous malformations or in some tumors. Collateral flow patterns may be identified in instances of thrombosis of major arteries, for example, utilization of the external carotid and ophthalmic arteries in cases of internal carotid artery occlusion; diminution or absence of flow is of course found distal to the site of the vascular occlusion itself. A general slowing of the circulation may be noted when the intracranial pressure is elevated, for whatever reason.

## COMPUTERIZED TOMOGRAPHY

It is difficult to overestimate the significance and impact of computerized tomographic (CT) scanning. With little or no hazard to the patient the CT scan permits remarkable assessment of the cranial and orbital contents, far beyond any previously attainable during life. Indeed, the advent of this technique has revolutionized the diagnostic approach to the neurologic patient. In brief, the scan furnishes important information under several circumstances: (1) when there is modification in the neural parenchyma itself, as evidenced by alterations in tissue density; (2) when there is change in the size or configuration of the ventricles; (3) when the supporting or vascular structures are altered; (4) when extraneous material such as blood or calcium is present. In neuro-ophthalmologic problems, alterations in the globe, the optic nerve, and the orbital contents are all displayed with remarkable clarity (See Fig. 4-20).

*Image enhancement* that utilizes intravenous iodinated contrast media is often desirable, especially in instances of neoplasm, aneurysm, or vascular malformation. Enhancement may assist in distinguishing between tumor and infarction; however, enhancement, presumably reflecting changes in the blood-brain barrier, may also appear within a softening (paralleling the uptake visible on an ordinary static isotopic scan). Such enhancement is not without risk. Idiosyncratic reactions to the iodinated dye occur, ranging from nausea, vomiting, and urticaria to bronchospasm, facial or glottal edema, pulmonary edema, syncope, coma, convulsions, cardiac arrhythmias, and cardiac arrest. These side effects generally develop within minutes of the injection. They are unpredictable, do not appear to be dose-related, and are not necessarily dependent on prior exposure to the dye. They tend to be more common in patients with known allergies, especially asthmatics. Pretesting appears to be of no real value; pretreatment of allergic individuals with antihistamines or corticosteriods is advocated, but with uncertain success. A history of prior major adverse reaction to iodinated dyes is a major contraindication to contrast enhancement.

Utilizing contemporary CT scanning techniques, views are obtained in a horizontal projection based on a line connecting the floor of the orbit and the external auditory meatus (Reid's line) (Fig. 4-15). Images so obtained (Fig. 4-16) are ordinarily easily understood in an anatomic sense. With early CT technology, the use of a semihorizontal projection tilted from the horizontal by as much as 20° resulted in images somewhat dis-

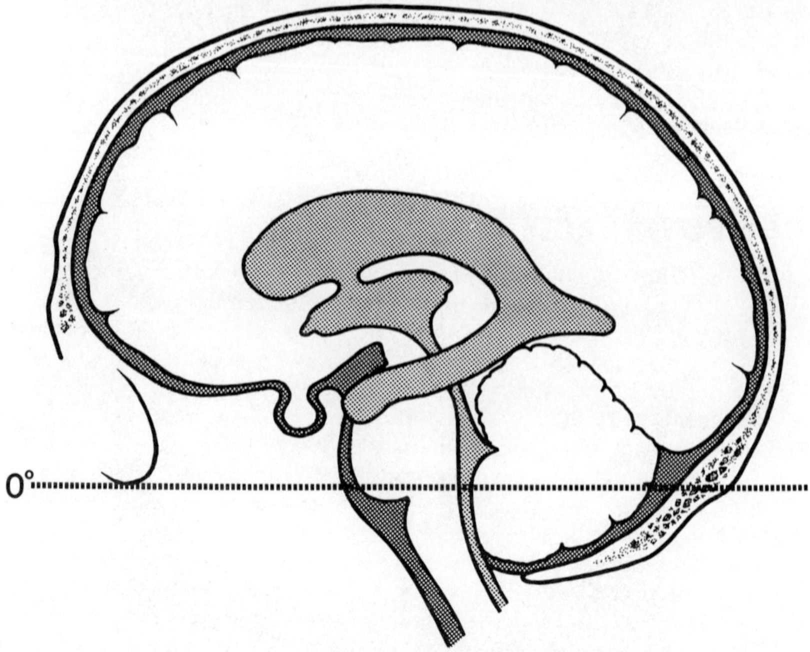


**FIGURE 4-15.** A horizontal projection based on Reid's line as used in contemporary CT scanning. (Modified from Hanaway and Strother.)

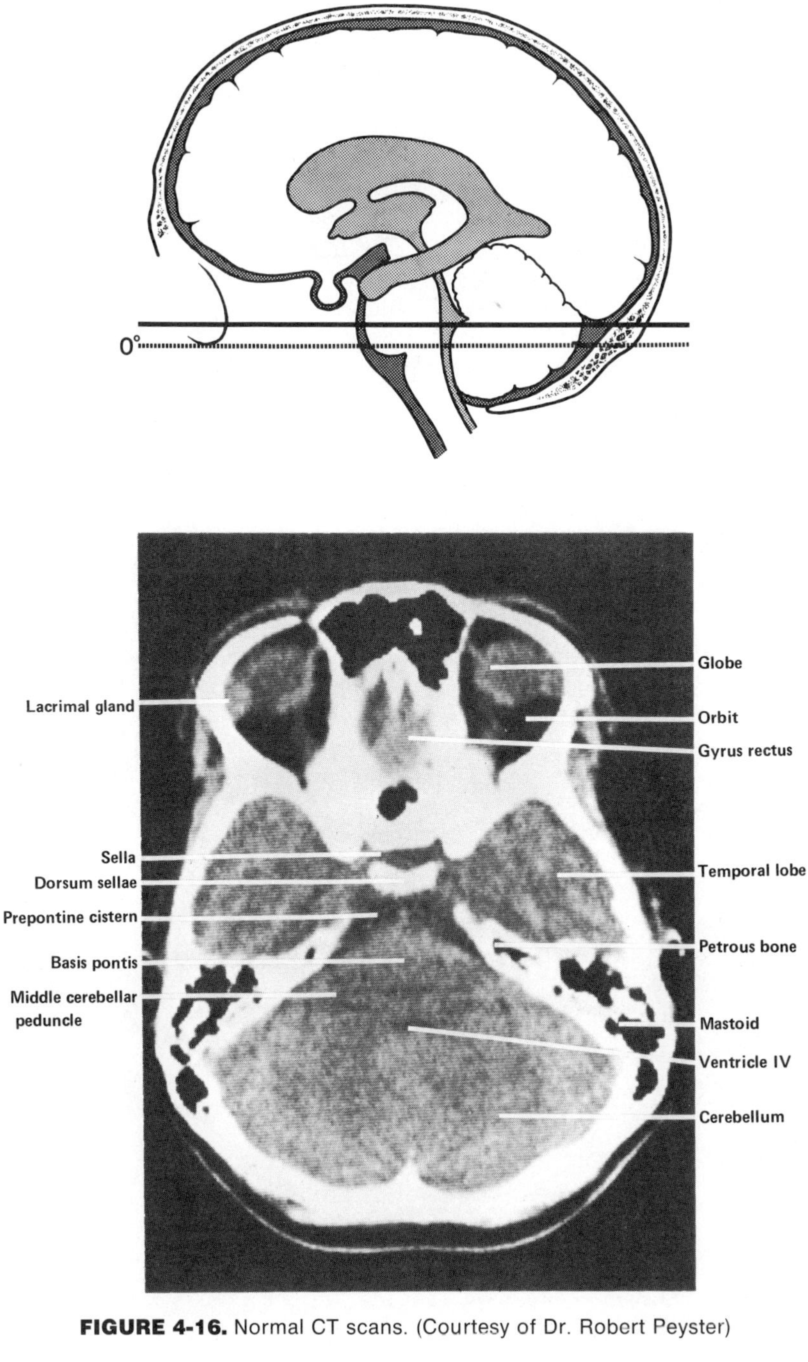


**FIGURE 4-16.** Normal CT scans. (Courtesy of Dr. Robert Peyster)

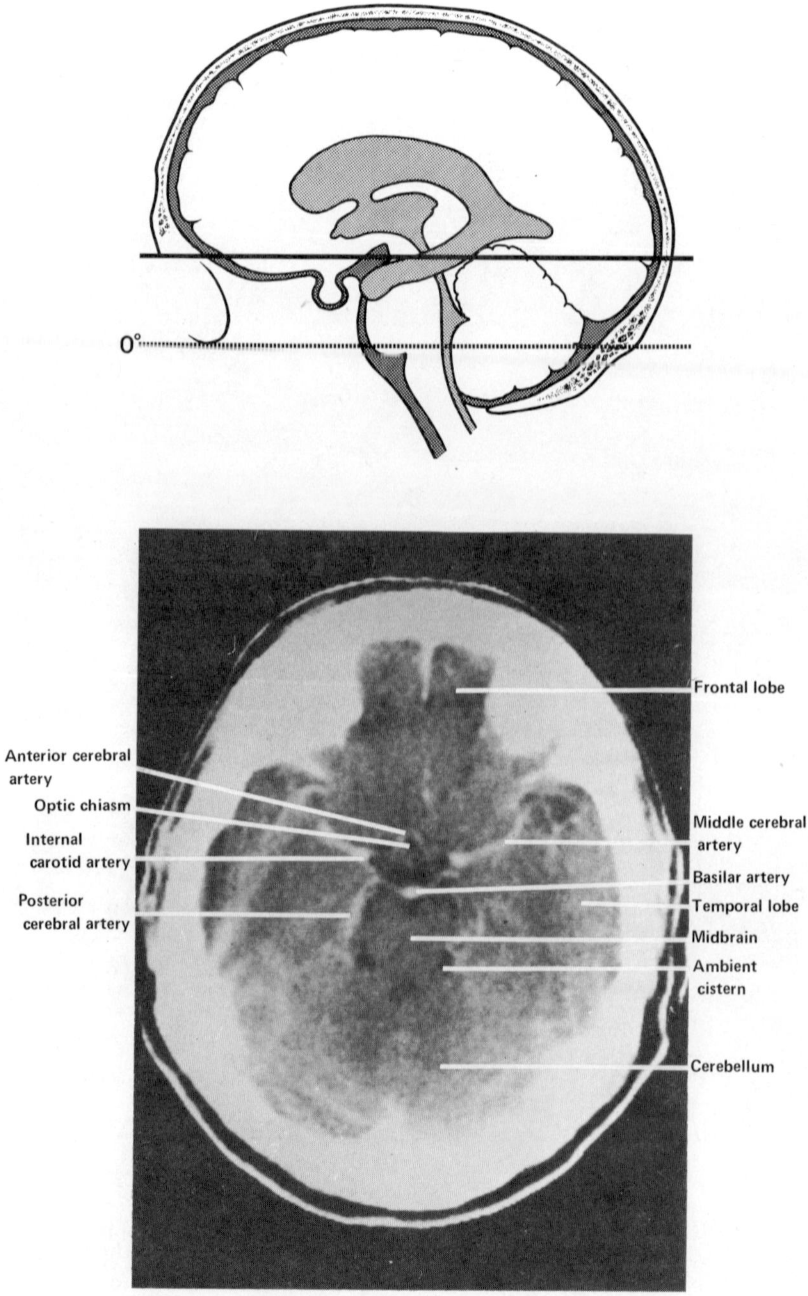


**FIGURE 4-16** *(continued).*

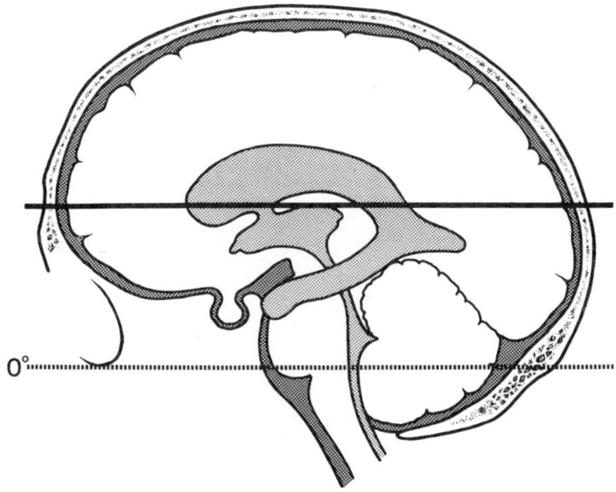


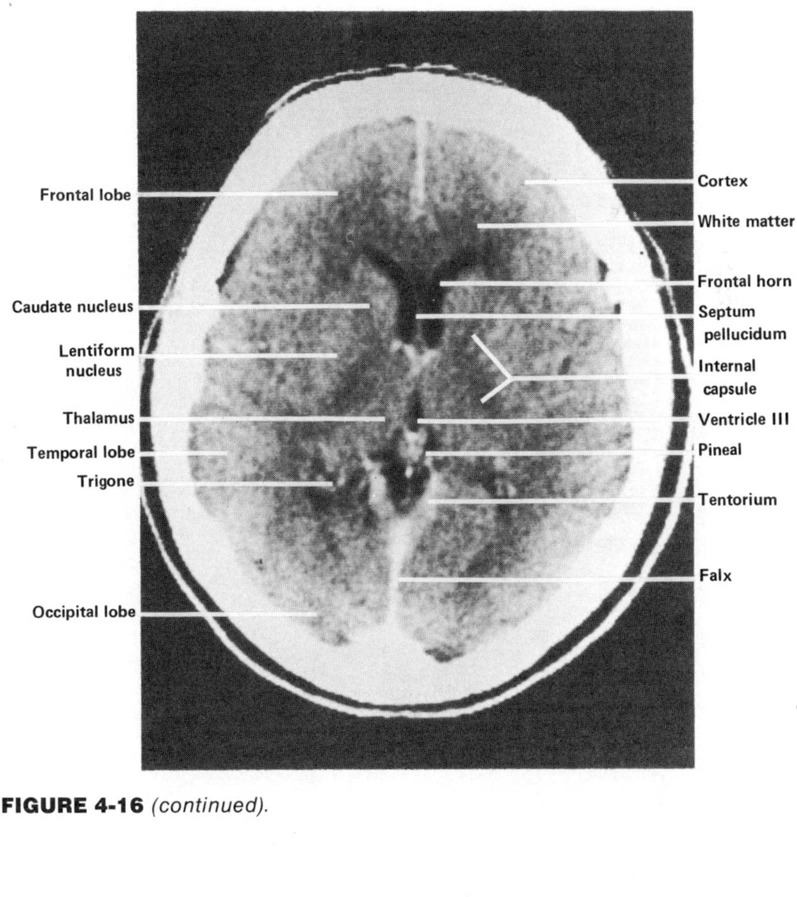


**FIGURE 4-16** *(continued).*

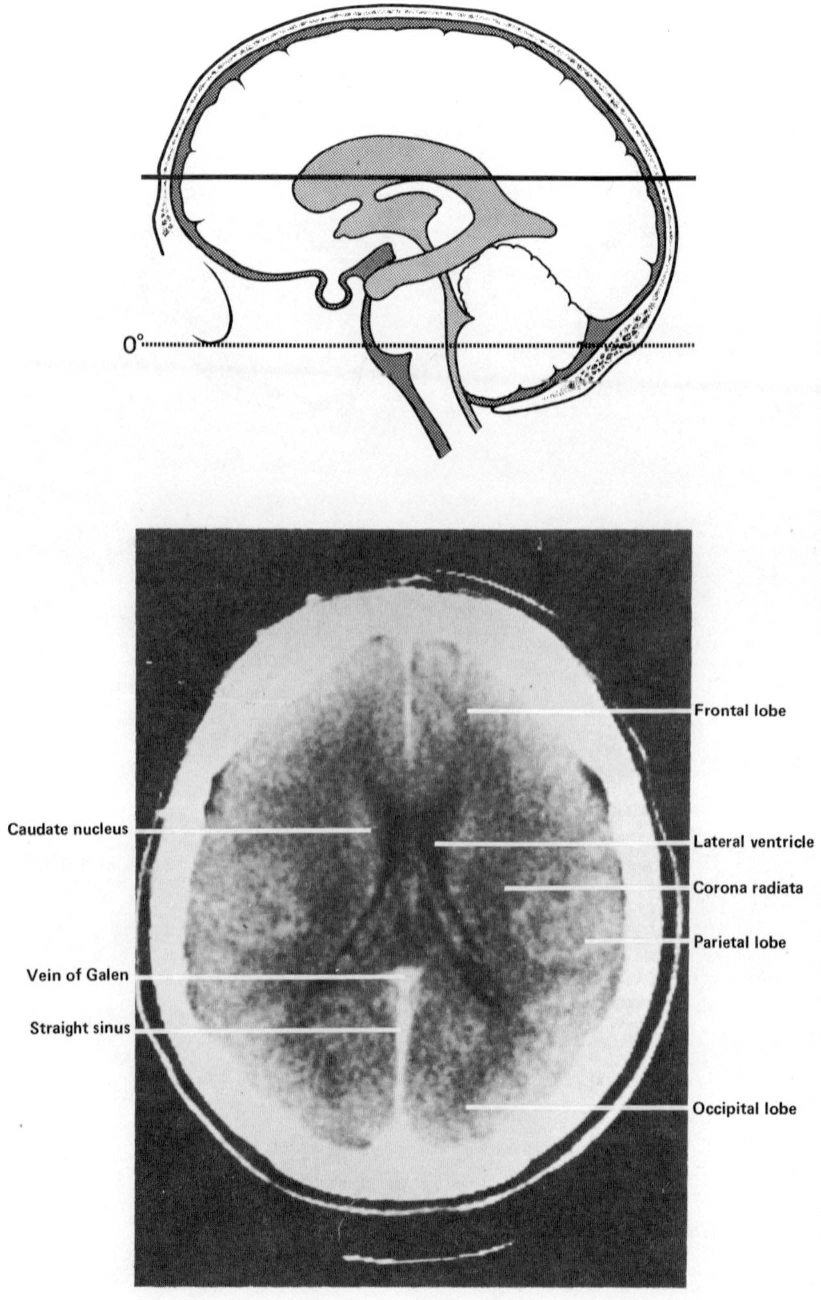


**FIGURE 4-16** *(continued).*

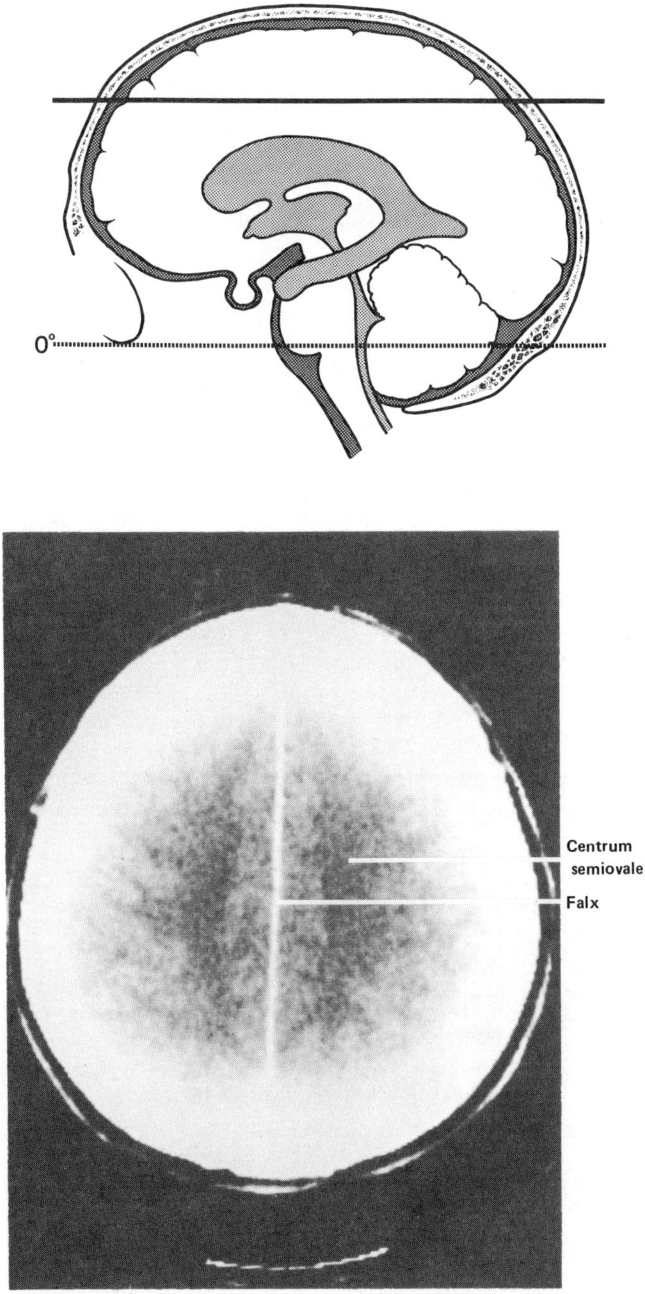


**FIGURE 4-16** *(continued).*

torted and at times difficult to interpret for the average observer. Computer-generated coronal and sagittal images provide substantial supplemental information in selected cases.

The CT scan finds application in virtually all types of neurologic patients. The ease with which the test is performed, the lack of major side effects, and its noninvasive character encourage its use from earliest infancy to old age. The diagnostic yield of the procedure is remarkable in a host of neurologic disorders. For example, an unsuspected vascular malformation, neoplasm, or porencephalic cyst may be demonstrated in a patient experiencing headaches, even in the face of a normal neurologic examination, and malformation, tumor, or focal atrophy may be visualized in individuals with seizures, especially when of a focal nature. In the demented individual the observation of gray or white matter degeneration, with or without ventricular enlargement, may prove of major diagnostic assistance in disorders as diverse as Alzheimer's disease or the leukodystrophies. Numerous examples of this sort can be cited. It must be emphasized, however, that the CT scan is of maximal benefit in cases screened and selected on the basis of relevant clinical presentation and reasonable diagnostic suspicion. The performance of CT scans as a matter of routine in all patients with complaints in or around the head is illogical and wasteful. The scan should properly be looked upon as a supplemental step in the diagnostic process; it follows a careful clinical appraisal and takes its place with, but not necessarily supplants, other noninvasive studies. In the final analysis, selection of cases on the basis of clinical assessment and judgment is critical to the rational application of this procedure.

In an attempt to clarify the indications for CT scanning in a variety of clinical settings, specific categories of neurologic disease may be considered:

## Cerebrovascular Disease

Diagnosis of *occlusive* cerebrovascular disease, whether thrombotic or embolic, is materially assisted by the CT scan (Fig. 4-17). An area of tissue ischemia and infarction may be recognized within relatively few hours of onset. As the lesion evolves, its appearance with the CT scan changes; in old infarcts, secondary effects such as localized ventricular dilatation become apparent. With embolic occlusion, a hemorrhagic infarction is ordinarily readily appreciated. Recognizable changes are dependent entirely on the presence of ischemic parenchymatous alterations. The patient with transient ischemic attacks (TIA) alone has as a matter of definition no fixed structural lesions and thus should evidence no appreciable change with the CT scan.

The CT scan is most informative in cerebral *hemorrhage* (Fig. 4-17). Even small amounts of blood within the parenchyma, or in the ventricles or subarachnoid space, can be identified with ease. An accurate delineation of an intracerebral hemorrhage is not simply an academic exercise: cerebellar hemorrhages, often difficult to diagnose clinically, are readily identified, thus permitting early, life-saving surgical intervention. In primary subarachnoid hemorrhage, CT scanning demonstrates blood in the subarachnoid space at the base, over the convexities, or between the hemispheres. With contrast enhancement, the underlying aneurysm or malformation may be highlighted. The course of the patient with a subarachnoid hemorrhage may also be monitored with a CT scan: resolution of blood, rebleeding, the parenchymatous effects of protracted spasm, and the development of obstructive hydrocephalus are all readily identified, permitting vigorous and early therapeutic intervention as indicated.

## Trauma

CT scanning is critical to the evaluation of the patient with craniocerebral trauma. It may provide important information as to the presence and extent of an extracerebral (epidural, subdural) clot and the degree of compression and shift of the underlying brain. An occasional extracerebral hematoma is isodense, however, and thus not evident with CT; isotopic brain scan and/or angiography are necessary for accurate diagnosis in such instances. Traumatic subarachnoid or intracerebral bleeding is ordinarily well visualized. A curious time lag may be noted between the traumatic incident itself and the appearance of an intracerebral hematoma on CT scanning; if such bleeding is suspected clinically, a repeat scan must be performed within a short period of time. Traumatic cerebral edema is well visualized, as are most contusions, although small contusion foci, particularly those placed inferiorly, may not be visualized. The CT scan also provides useful information regarding late effects of trauma such as normal pressure hydrocephalus, brain abscess, or porencephalic cyst. Patients with the common postconcussive syndrome, including headache, impaired concentration and memory, impotence, depression, and vertigo, usually have normal CT scans.

## Tumors

The CT scan is of great help in the identification of both primary and metastatic intracranial tumors, often very early in the clinical course. The location of the neoplasm, its size, its effect on adjacent parenchyma, and even its specific histologic type may all be deduced from the CT scan, particularly when enhancement is employed (Fig. 4-18). The scan may also provide very early evidence of uncal herniation. The course of a patient receiving radiation therapy may be followed easily with this technique; changes in tumor size and evidence of radiation necrosis are ordinarily easily identified.

The CT scan is also important in instances of *pseudotumor cerebri*

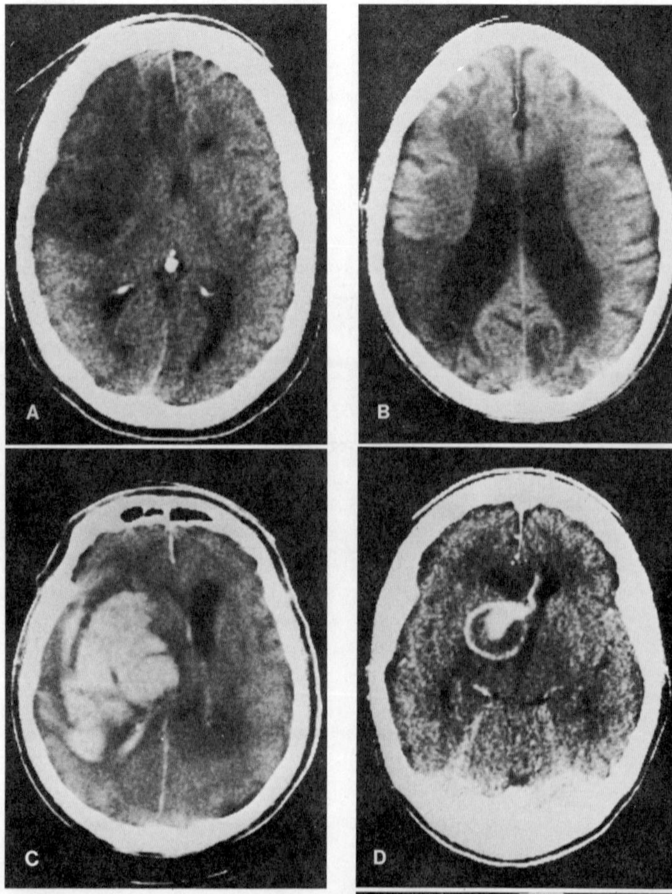


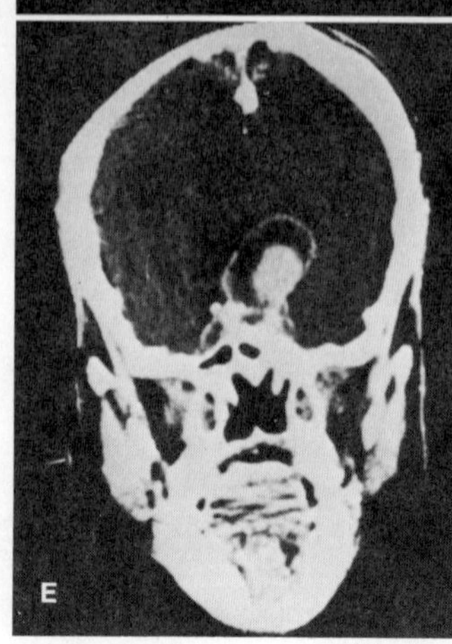


**FIGURE 4-17.** Recent *(A)* and old *(B)* infarctions, both in distribution of the middle cerebral artery. In the former, marked edema with ventricular shift is evident. *C,* Hypertensive intracerebral hemorrhage of massive proportions, in a typical ganglionic distribution. There is striking compression and shift of the ventricles; a small amount of blood is visible within the ventricular system. *D* and *E,* Large congenital intracracial aneurysm as seen in horizontal and coronal projections. (Courtesy of Dr. Robert Peyster)

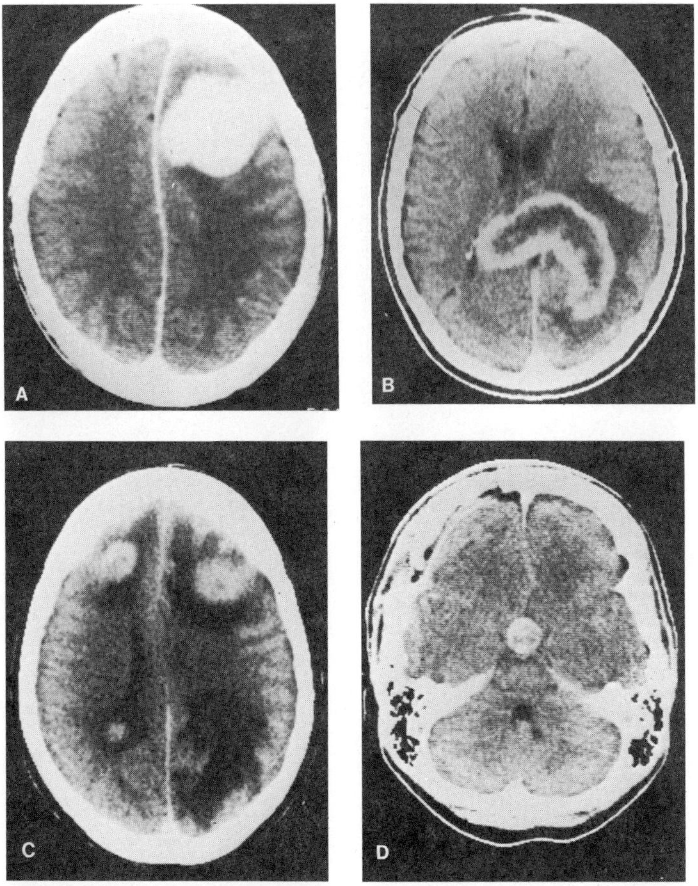

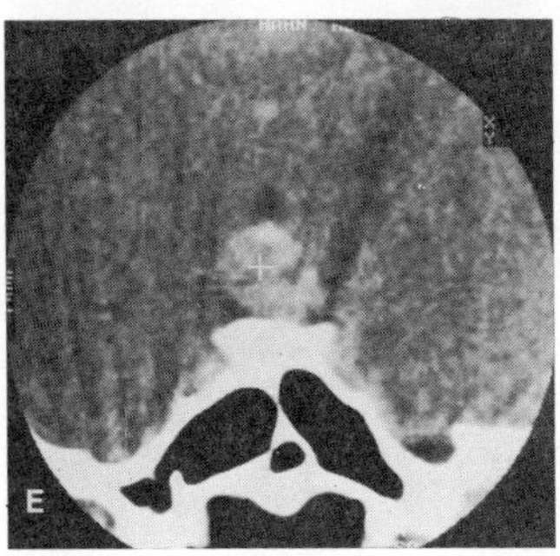

**FIGURE 4-18.** Frontal convexity meningioma *(A)* and malignant glioma of the corpus callosum *(B)*, both demonstrating striking contrast enhancement. *C*, Metastatic bronchogenic carcinoma. Multiple lesions are associated with considerable edema. *D* and *E*, Craniopharyngioma as visualized in horizontal and coronal scans. (Courtesy of Dr. Robert Peyster)

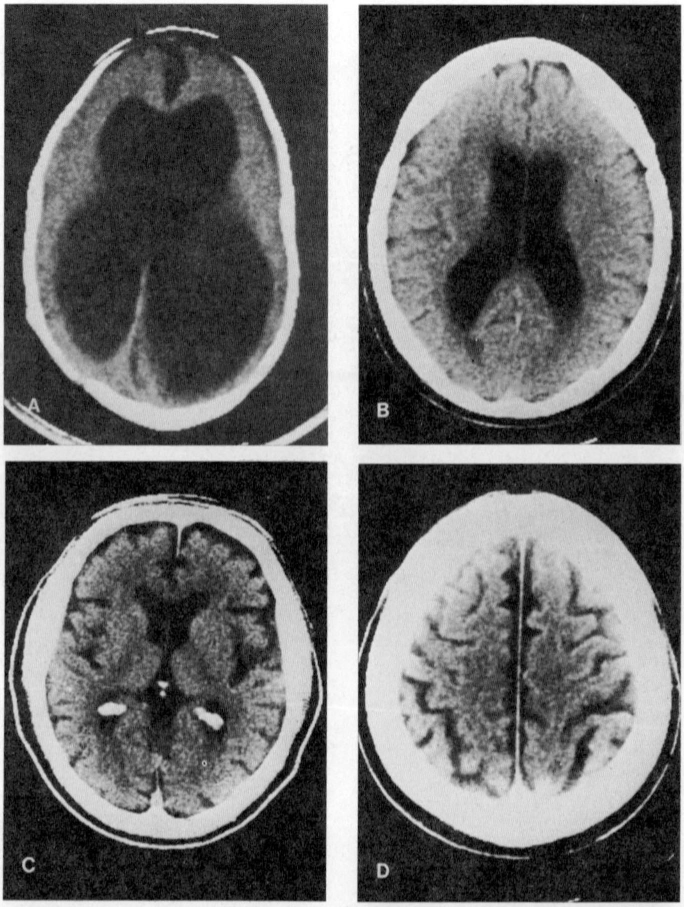


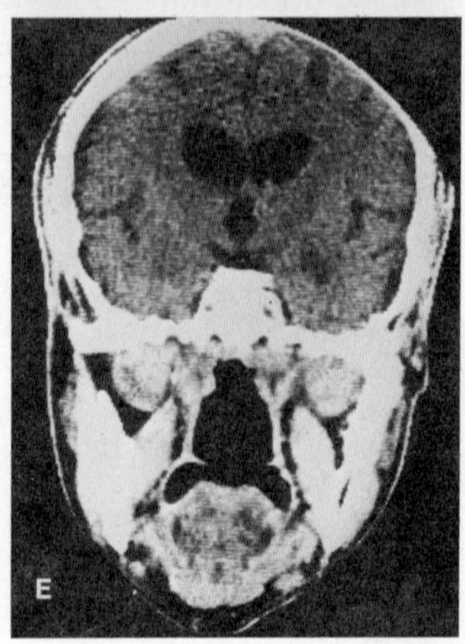


**FIGURE 4-19.** *A,* Obstructive hydrocephalus in a case of Arnold-Chiari malformation. *B,* Normal pressure hydrocephalus, demonstrating ventricular enlargement with no significant cortical atrophy. At other levels, periventricular low absorption is found. *C* and *D,* Alzheimer's disease. Enlargement of ventricles is associated with marked atrophy of the cortical mantle. *E,* Huntington's disease. Atrophy of the caudate nuclei is well seen in the coronal CT projection; moderate cortical atrophy is evident as well. (Courtesy of Dr. Robert Peyster)

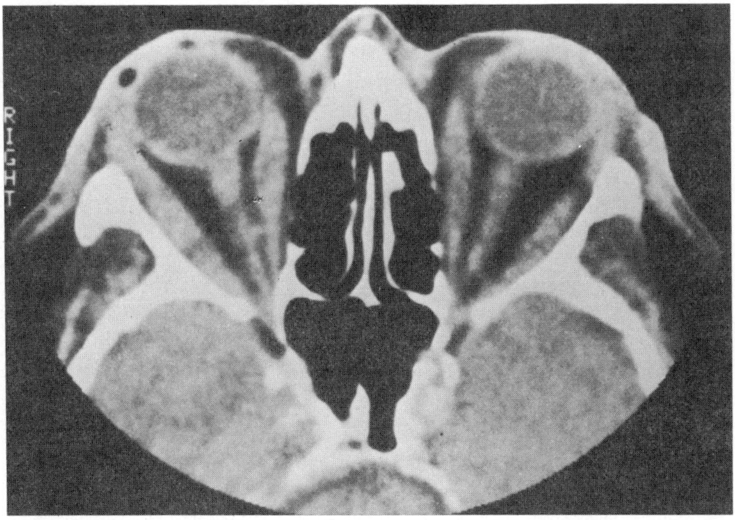


**FIGURE 4-20.** Thyrotoxic ophthalmopathy. There is bilateral proptosis with asymmetric enlargement of the medial and lateral recti and of the optic nerves. (Courtesy of Dr. Robert Peyster)

(benign intracranial hypertension). This disorder is characterized clinically by signs of increased intracranial pressure without evidence of focal brain disease and appears under circumstances as diverse as obesity, pregnancy, hypothyroidism, vitamin A intoxication, or prior use of antibiotics such as tetracycline. The brain is swollen, but the ventricles are normal or reduced in size and in normal position. In the past, ventriculography and/or angiography were necessary to exclude a deep midline space-occupying lesion under such circumstances; at present, CT scan provides the required information rapidly and without risk to the patient. Serial scans may assist in determining the efficacy of treatment.

## Degenerative Disorders

Since many degenerative, or heredodegenerative, disorders are characterized by systematic degeneration of the cerebral gray matter, the CT scan may be remarkably informative (Fig. 4-19). For example, in diffuse degenerations of the cortex such as Alzheimer's disease, shrinkage of the cortical mantle and compensatory enlargement of the ventricles *(hydrocephalus ex vacuo)* are visualized. In contrast, the rare case of Pick's disease exhibits atrophic changes restricted to the frontal and temporal poles. The distinction between Alzheimer's disease and normal pressure hydrocephalus (NPH) is of major importance therapeutically, and here the CT scan is of decided assistance; in contrast to the changes of Alzheimer's disease, the ventricles in NPH are enlarged but the cortex little atrophied if at all. There is some question, however, as to whether the CT scan alone can be accepted as the sole definitive diagnostic procedure in such cases, and other tests, in particular isotope cisternography, may be required before surgical intervention is contemplated.

Of the heredodegenerative diseases involving the basal ganglia, the CT scan demonstrates enlargement of the ventricles and cortical atrophy, and, at times, shrinkage of the caudate nuclei in Huntington's disease. In other disorders of the basal ganglia such as Parkinson's disease the scan is of little or no assistance. In the spinocerebellar degenerations, CT scanning may demonstrate atrophy of the cerebellar cortex or of the major surrounding structures such as the basis pontis; the scan is of little benefit in those instances in which the disease is predominantly spinal (e.g., Friedreich's ataxia). In the motor system diseases, for example, amyotrophic lateral sclerosis, the CT scan has no significant role.

## Other Neurologic Diseases

The CT scan offers striking assistance in the diagnosis and management of *brain abscess.* In the early stage of abscess formation, so-called acute cerebritis, the changes are nonspecific and difficult to interpret. As the abscess evolves, however, the changes are readily recognized; shrinkage of the cavity and subsidence of edema are effectively monitored, with important therapeutic implications. The scan is of little help in most other intracranial infectious processes, although in intensely necrotizing viral encephalitides, such as herpes simplex encephalitis, focal softening or hemorrhage may be observed.

Utilizing enhancement techniques, CT scanning may demonstrate the lesions (plaques) of multiple sclerosis if they are sufficiently large. Ventricular enlargement may be encountered in long-standing cases. The presence of widespread white matter degeneration is readily recognized in classic Schilder's disease and in a variety of leukodystrophies. The scan is of negligible significance in metabolic encephalopathy. Brain edema may appear in disorders such as acute lead intoxication; cortical atrophy may be seen as a residual of anoxic or hypoglycemic encephalopathy.

CT scanning also has broad applicability in the neurologic assessment of the infant and child. Ventricular dilatation, calcification, cyst formation, or multicystic degeneration may provide evidence of congenital infection or of birth trauma or hypoxia. Intraventricular hemorrhage is commonly seen in premature infants with severe respiratory distress. Scanning, especially sequentially performed, is informative in the evaluation of infants who fail to thrive or those with developmental delay or intellectual retardation, and in those with progressive enlargement of the head. The scan is of value in following the course of ventricular enlargement in hydrocephalics and is in fact a more reliable guide than simple measurement of increasing head size alone. The efficacy of shunting procedures, and the appearance of shunt malfunction and failure are readily monitored postoperatively.

Numerous developmental anomalies may also be identified with the CT scan, such as cerebral or cerebellar hypoplasia and agenesis of the corpus callosum. Ballooning of the fourth ventricle is easily seen in the Dandy-Walker syndrome. Among the phakomatoses (neuroectodermal dysplasias), patients with tuberous sclerosis exhibit subependymal calcifications and periventricular masses ("tubers"), occasionally with gliomatous degeneration, and superficial vascular anomalies may appear in the Sturge-Weber syndrome. Individuals with von Hippel-Lindau disease may also exhibit vascular malformations, especially in the cerebellum, and in neurofibromatosis (von Recklinghausen's disease) the CT scan may demonstrate intracranial neoplasms such as optic glioma, glioblastoma, or acoustic neurinoma.

## BIBLIOGRAPHY


Callaway, E., Tueting, P., and Koslow, S. H. (eds.): *Event-Related Brain Potentials in Man.* Academic Press, New York, 1978.

Cohen, H. L., and Brumlik, J.: *A Manual of Electromyography.* Harper & Row, New York, 1968.

Croll, M. N., Brady, L. W., Faust, D. S., et al.: *Comparison brain scanning with mercury 203 and technetium* $^{99}$m. Radiology 90:747, 1968.

Davidoff, L. M., and Dyke, C. G.: *The Normal Encephalogram.* Lea & Febiger, Philadelphia, 1951.

Davidoff, L. M., and Epstein, B. S.: *The Abnormal Pneumoencephalogram.* Lea & Febiger, Philadelphia, 1955.

Fishman, R. A.: *Cerebrospinal Fluid in Diseases of the Nervous System.* W. B. Saunders Co., Philadelphia, 1980.

Gibbs, F. A., and Gibbs, E. L.: *Atlas of Electroencephalography.* Addison-Wesley Publishing Co., Reading, Mass., 1950–1964, vol. 1-3.

Gutterman, P., and Shenkin, H. A.: *Cerebral scans in completed strokes: value in prognosis of clinical course.* J.A.M.A. 207:145, 1969.

Hanaway, J., Scott, W. R., and Strother, C. M.: *Atlas of the Human Brain and the Orbit for Computed Tomography.* ed. 2. Warren H. Green, Inc., St. Louis, 1980.

Kiloh, L. G., McComas, A. J., and Osselton, J. W.: *Clinical Electroencephalography.* ed. 3. Butterworths, London, 1972.

Klass, D. W., and Daly, D. D. (eds.): *Current Practice of Clinical Electroencephalography.* Raven Press, New York, 1979.

Kooi, K. A., Tucker, R. P., and Marshall, R. E.: *Fundamentals of Electroencephalography.* ed. 2. Harper & Row, Hagerstown, Md., 1978.

Ledley, R. S., DiChiro, G., Luessenhop, A. J., et al.: *Computerized transaxial x-ray tomography of the human body.* Science 186:207, 1974.

Lenman, J. A. R., and Ritchie, A. E.: *Clinical Electromyography.* ed. 2. Pitman Medical and Scientific Publishing Co., London, 1977.

Lennox, W. G.: *Epilepsy and Related Disorders.* Little, Brown and Co., Boston, 1960.

Matsui, T., and Hirano, A.: *An Atlas of the Human Brain for Computerized Tomography.* Sgaku-Shoin, Ltd., Tokyo, 1978.

Matthews, W. B., Small, D. G., Small, M., et al.: *Pattern reversal evoked visual potential in the diagnosis of multiple sclerosis.* J. Neurol. Neurosurg. Psychiatry 40:1009-1014, 1977.

New, P. F. J., and Scott, W. R.: *Computed Tomography of the Brain and Orbit (EMI Scanning).* Williams & Wilkins Co., Baltimore, 1975.

New, P. F. J., Scott, W. R., Schnur, J. A., et al.: *Computerized axial tomography with the EMI scanner.* Radiology 110:109, 1974.

Robertson, E. G.: *Pneumoencephalography.* Charles C Thomas, Springfield, Ill., 1967.

Schneck, S. A., and Claman, H. N.: *CSF immunoglobulins in multiple sclerosis and other neurological diseases.* Arch. Neurol. 20:132, 1969.

Silverman, D., Saunders, M. G., Schwab, R. S., et al.: *Cerebral death and the electroencephalogram.* J.A.M.A. 209:1505, 1969.

Starr, A.: *Sensory evoked potentials in clinical disorders of the nervous system.* Ann. Rev. Neuroscience, 1:103-127, 1978.

Taveras, J. M., and Wood, E. H.: *Diagnostic Neuroradiology.* Williams & Wilkins Co., Baltimore, 1964.

Toole, J. F. (ed.): *Special Techniques for Neurologic Diagnosis.* F. A. Davis Co., Philadelphia, 1969.

Uemura, T., Suzuki, J., Hozawa, J., et al.: *Neuro-Otological Examination.* University Park Press, Baltimore, 1977.

Wickbom, I.: *Angiography of the carotid artery, Parts 1 and 2.* Acta Radiol. (Suppl.) (Stockh.) 72, 1948.

Williams, R. L. and Karacan, I.: *Sleep Disorders, Diagnosis and Treatment.* John Wiley and Sons, New York, 1978.

# Appendix

## MUSCLE INNERVATION

*(After Raezer)*

ORDER OF ARRANGEMENT: *Muscle action; muscles with spinal cord segments* (C—cervical, T—thoracic, L—lumbar, S—sacral); *cord of plexus —peripheral nerve.* Asterisks (*) indicate the muscles chiefly responsible for the movement in question.

UPPER EXTREMITY—BRACHIAL PLEXUS—C5 to T1

1. FLEXORS AND LATERAL ROTATORS OF HEAD:
   *a. Sternocleidomastoid m.—medulla and C2, C3, C4—Cranial Nerve XI
   b. Posterior neck m.—C2, C3, C4 and nerves
      i Longus capitis
      ii Rectus capitis anterior
      iii Longus colli
2. EXTENSORS OF HEAD:
   a. Trapezius m.—medulla and C2, C3, C4—Cranial Nerve XI
   b. Posterior neck m.—C2, C3, C4 and nerves
      *i Longissimus capitis
      ii Semispinalis capitis

3. Elevators of shoulders: Test: Shrugging of shoulders
   *a. Trapezius m.—same as 2a
   b. Elevators of scapula—C3, C4, C5—dorsal scapular n.
      i Levator scapulae
      ii Rhomboidei

4. Retractors of shoulders:
   *a. Trapezius m.—same as 2a
   b. Rhomboidei—same as 3b

5. Lateral abductors of arm: *Above 90° angle* (also fix scapula below 90°)
   a. Trapezius m.—same as 2a
   b. Anterior serratus m.—C5, C6, C7—long thoracic n.

6. Forward thrusting of arm: Test: Patient extends arms forward placing the palms against a wall and pushes body toward the wall keeping the arms extended. Examiner observes scapula for "winging" (separation of scapula from back) with the inferior angle of the scapula pulled up and in
   a. Anterior serratus m.—same as 5b

7. Adductors of humerus:
   *a. Latissimus dorsi m.—C6, C7, C8—posterior cord of brachial plexus—thoracodorsal n.
   *b. Pectoralis major m.—C5 to T1—lateral and medial cords—anterior thoracic n.
   c. Teres major m.—C5, C6—posterior cord—subscapularis n.
   d. Teres minor m.—C5, C6—posterior cord—axillary n.
   e. Coracobrachialis m.—C5, C6—musculocutaneous n.

8. Flexors of humerus: Test: Arm at side pushing forward against resistance—"punching" action
   *a. Pectoralis major and minor m.—same as 7b
   b. Deltoid m.—C5, C6—axillary n.
   c. Subscapularis m.—C5, C6—posterior cord—subscapularis n.
   d. Coracobrachialis m.—same as 7e

9. Extensors or retractors of arm: Test: Arm and elbow at side pushing back against resistance—"swimming" action
   *a. Latissimus dorsi m.—Same as 7a

10. Abductors of arm: Test: Arm laterally abducted *up to 90° angle*
   a. Initiator of abduction—C5, C6—suprascapular n.
      i Supraspinatus m.
   *b. Deltoid m.—same as 8b

11. Muscles of respiration:
   a. *Normal respiration:*
      i Diaphragm—C3, C4, C5—phrenic n.

- ii Intercostals
- iii Subcostals
- iv Levator costarum

(ii–iv: T1 to T12—intercostal n.)

- v Scaleni—C4, C5—cervical nerves

b. *Accessory muscles of respiration:*
- i Sternocleidomastoid m.—same as 1a
- ii Trapezius m.—Same as 2a
- iii Anterior serratus m.—same as 5b
- iv Latissimus dorsi m. (coughing)—same as 7a
- v Pectoralis major and minor—same as 7b
- vi Rhomboidei m.—same as 3b
- vii Supraspinatus m.—same as 10a

12. MEDIAL OR INWARD ROTATORS OF ARM: Test: Arm extended at side and rotated inward against resistance:
   a. Pectoralis major m.—same as 7b
   b. Latissimus dorsi m.—same as 7a
   c. Teres major m.—same as 7c
   d. Subscapularis m.—same as 8c
   e. Deltoid m.—same as 8b

13. LATERAL OR OUTWARD ROTATORS OF ARM: Test: Arm held at side and laterally rotated against resistance:
   a. Teres minor m.—same as 7d
   b. Infraspinatus m.—same as 10a
   c. Deltoid m.—same as 8b

14. FLEXORS OF FOREARM (elbow):
   a. *Chief flexors:* C5, C6—lateral cord—musculocutaneous n.
      - *i Biceps brachii
      - ii Brachialis
      - iii Coracobrachialis
   b. *Accessory flexors:*
      - i Brachioradialis—C5, C6—posterior cord—radial n.
      - ii Pronator teres—C6—median n.
      - iii Palmaris longus—C6—median n.

15. EXTENSORS OF FOREARM (elbow):
   a. Triceps brachii m.—C6, C7, C8—posterior cord—radial n.
   b. Anconeus—same as triceps

16. PRONATORS OF FOREARM (rotation of forearm inward):
   a. Pronator teres—C6—median n.
   b. Pronator quadratus—C7, C8—median n.
   c. Flexor carpi radialis—same as pronator teres

17. SUPINATORS OF FOREARM (rotation of forearm outward):
   a. *Supinator m.:* C5, C6—posterior cord—radial n. (arm extended)

b. *Biceps brachii:* Same as 4a (arm flexed)

18. Flexors of wrist:
    a. *Main flexors:* C6 – median n.
        i Flexor carpi radialis
        ii Palmaris longus
        iii Flexor digitorum sublimis
    b. *Accessory flexion:*
        i Flexor carpi ulnaris – C8, T1 – ulnar n.
        ii Flexor digitorum profundus – C8, T1 – median and ulnar n.

19. Extensors of wrist: All innervated by C6, C7, C8 – radial n.
    a. Extensor carpi radialis longus } extend wrist
    b. Extensor carpi radialis brevis } extend wrist
    c. Extensor digitorum communis – extends all phalanges of fingers
    d. Extensor digiti quinti proprius – extends phalanges of little finger
    e. Extensor carpi ulnaris – extends ulnar side of wrist
    f. Extensor pollicis brevis – extends proximal phalanx of thumb
    g. Extensor pollicis longus – extends distal phalanx of thumb
    h. Extensor indicis proprius – extends index finger

20. Adductors of wrist: Movement of wrist toward the ulna
    a. Flexor carpi ulnaris – same as 18b
    b. Extensor carpi ulnaris – same as 19e

21. Abductors of wrist:
    a. *Flexor carpi radialis:* Same as 18a
    b. *Extensors that abduct:* Same as 19
        i Extensor carpi radialis longus and brevis
        ii Extensor pollicis longus and brevis
    c. *Abductor pollicis longus* (abductor of base of thumb): C6, C7, C8 – radial n.

## HAND

I. Movements of thumb:
    1. *Abduction of thumb:*
        a. Abductor pollicis brevis (abducts first metacarpal) – C6, C7 – median n.
        b. Abductor pollicis longus – C6, C7, C8 – radial n.
    2. *Extensors of thumb:* C6, C7, C8 – radial n.
        a. Extensor pollicis longus and brevis
    3. *Adductor of thumb:* (pure adduction of thumb when thumb is on a plane with the hand)
        a. Adductor pollicis – C8, T1 – ulnar n.
    4. *Flexor of thumb:* C6, C7 – median n.
        a. Proximal phalanx – flexor pollicis brevis

b. Terminal phalanx—flexor pollicis longus

5. *Opposition of thumb to fingers:* C6, C7—median n.
   a. Opponens pollicis—assisted by
      i Flexor pollicis brevis—4a
      ii Adductor pollicis—3

II. MOVEMENTS OF SMALL FINGER: C8, T1—ulnar n.

1. *Abductor of little finger:*
   a. Abductor digiti quinti
2. *Flexor of little finger:*
   a. Flexor digiti quinti
3. *Opposition of little finger to thumb:*
   a. Opponens digiti quinti

N.B. All 3 of the above muscles act only on the metacarpophalangeal joint

III. MOVEMENTS OF FINGERS:

1. *Flexor of metacarpophalangeal joints:* C8—median n.
   a. Flexor digitorum sublimis
2. *Flexor of distal interphalangeal joints:* C7 to T1—median and ulnar n.
   a. Flexor dignitorum profundus
3. *Extensor of all joints of 4 fingers:* C6, C7, C8—radial n.
   a. Extensor digitorum profundus
   b. Extensor digiti quinti proprius
   c. Extensor indicis proprius
4. *Accessory extensors of interphalangeal joints and flexors of metacarpophalangeal joints*
   a. Lateral 2 lumbricales—C7 to T1—median n.
   b. Medial 2 lumbricales—C8, T1—ulnar n.
   c. Interossei m.—C8, T1—ulnar n.
5. *Ab*ductors (spreading) and *ad*ductors (approximating) of fingers —C8, T1—ulnar n.
   a. Interossei m.
      i 4 volar interossei *ad*duct
      ii 4 dorsal interossei *ab*duct
6. *Thenar eminence of hand:* Muscles at base of thumb—C6, C7, C8, T1
7. *Hypothenar eminence of hand:* Muscles at base of little finger—C8, T1

## SUMMARY OF MUSCLE INNERVATION UPPER EXTREMITY

1. All movements of head and neck are initiated through the medulla and C2, C3, and C4—cranial nerve XI and respective cervical nerves.

2. Shrugging and retraction of shoulders mediated through the me-

dulla and C2, C3, C4, and C5—cranial nerve XI and respective cervical nerves.

3. Paralysis of deltoid alone with normal flexion of wrist localizes the lesion to C5 segment.

4. Abduction and lateral rotation of arm, flexion of the elbow and supination of the forearm are all carried out through C5 and C6 segments *only*.

5. Flexion of metacarpophalangeal joints of the 4 fingers is mediated only by C6 segment.

6. Retraction of arm (swimming action) is initiated through C6, C7, and C8—thoracodorsal nerve.

7. Retraction of the arm, extension of the elbow, wrist and all the fingers, abduction of the wrist and thumb, and pronation of the forearm are all mediated through C6, C7, and C8 segments.

8. Flexion of the terminal phalanges of all 5 fingers is initiated through C7, C8, and T1 segments.

9. The muscles of the hypothenar eminence of the hand and interossei are innervated by C8 and T1 only through the ulnar nerve.

10. Adduction, flexion, and medial rotation of humerus initiated through C5 to T1 and all portions of the brachial plexus.

The ten summary movements noted above will be seen to follow a natural progression of movement. This will be made more clear if one performs these movements for oneself in the order in which they are written. Furthermore this will aid greatly in fixing the above pattern and make memorization less arduous.

It should be noted that No. 10 is a set of movements that include the whole brachial plexus and hence is always involved to a greater or lesser extent with any lesion of the brachial plexus, or cord segments from C5 to T1.

## LOWER EXTREMITY

### LUMBOSACRAL PLEXUS—L1 to S2

1. FLEXORS OF HIP JOINT: L2, L3 and L4
   - *a. Iliopsoas m.—L2, L3 and L4—ant. rami of L2, L3 and L4 and femoral n.
   - b. Rectus femoris, c. Pectineus m., d. Sartorius m. } L2, L3 and L4—femoral n.
   - e. *Ad*ductor longus and brevis, f. *Ab*ductor magnus, g. Obturator externus } L3 and L4—obturator n.

2. ADDUCTORS OF THIGH: L2, L3 and L4
   a. Adductor magnus
      i Adductor longus
      ii Adductor brevis
   b. Gracilis
   c. Obturator externus
   } L2, L3 and L4—obturator n.
   d. Sartorius m.
   e. Pectineus m.
   } L2, L3—femoral n.

3. EXTENSION OF KNEE: L3, L4 (±L5, S1)
   *a. Quadriceps femoris—L3, L4
   b. Tensor fasciae latae—L4 (L5 and S1)—superior gluteal n.

4. ABDUCTORS OF FEMUR: L4, L5, S1 (S2)
   a. Gluteus medius
   b. Gluteus minimus
   c. Tensor fasciae latae
   } L4, L5, S1—superior gluteal n.
   d. Superior and inferior gemelli m.
   e. Obturator internus m.
   f. Piriformis m.
   } S1, S2—anterior rami n.

5. EXTENSORS OF HIP:
   a. Gluteus maximus—L5, S1, S2—inferior gluteal n.
   b. Biceps femoris m.
   c. Semitendinosus m.
   d. Semimembranosus m.
   } L5, S1, S2—sciatic n.

6. LATERAL ROTATORS OF THIGH: L2 to S2
   a. Sartorius—same as 2d
   b. Adductor magnus, longus and brevis—same as 2a
   c. Obturator externus—same as 2c
   d. Gluteus maximus—same as 5a
   e. Biceps femoris (when knee is flexed)—same as 5b
   f. Inferior gemellus m.—same as 4d
   g. Piriformis m.—same as 4f
   h. Obturator internus m.—same as 4e
   i. Superior gemellus m.—same as 4d

7. MEDIAL ROTATORS OF FEMUR: L4, L5, S1
   a. Tensor fasciae latae—same as 3b
   b. Gluteus medius and minimus—same as 4a and 4b
   c. Adductor magnus m.—same as 2a

8. FLEXORS OF KNEE: L2 to S2
   a. Sartorius—same as 2d
   b. Gracilis—same as 2b
   c. Biceps femoris—same as 5b

d. Semitendinosus
e. Semimembranosus } same as 5c and 5d
f. Gastrocnemius – S1, S2 – tibial n.

9. DORSIFLEXORS OF ANKLE (foot): L4, L5, S1 – deep peroneal n.
   a. Tibialis anticus m.
   b. Extensor digitorum longus m.
   c. Peroneus tertius
   d. Extensor hallucis longus

10. EXTENSORS OF TOES: L4, L5 and S1 – deep peroneal n.
    a. Extensor digitorum longus and brevis
    b. Extensor hallucis longus

11. PLANTAR FLEXORS OF FOOT: L4, L5, S1, S2
    a. Peroneus longus and brevis – L4, L5, S1 – superficial peroneal n.
    b. Gastrocnemius m. – S1, S2 – tibial n.
    c. Soleus
    d. Flexor digitorum longus
    e. Flexor hallucis longus } L5, S1, S2 – tibial n.
    f. Tibialis posticus

12. INVERSION OF FOOT: L4, L5, S1
    a. Tibialis anticus – L4, L5, S1 – deep peroneal n.
    b. Tibialis posticus – L5, S1 – tibial n.

13. EVERSION OF FOOT: L4, L5, S1
    a. Peroneus tertius – L4, L5, S1 – *deep* peroneal n.
    b. Peroneus longus and brevis – L4, L5, S1 – *superficial* peroneal n.

14. MEDIAL ROTATORS OF FOOT (with knee flexed and foot flat on floor): L4 to S2
    a. Semitendinosus
    b. Semimembranosus } same as 5c and 5d
    c. Sartorius m.
    d. Gracilis m. } same as 2b and 2d
    e. Popliteus m. – L4, L5, S1 – tibial n.

15. LATERAL ROTATOR OF FOOT WITH KNEE FLEXED:
    a. Bicep femoris m. – L5, S1, S2 – Sciatic n.

16. PLANTAR FLEXORS OF TOES: L4 to S2
    a. Flexor digitorum longus
    b. Lumbricales (same action as in hand)
    c. Flexor hallucis longus } L5 to S2 – tibial n.
    d. *Ab*ductor hallucis longus
    e. Flexor digitorum brevis
    f. Flexor hallucis brevis } L4, L5, S1 – medial plantar n. – branch of tibial n.

g. Flexor digiti quinti brevis } S1, S2—lateral plantar n.
h. Interossei } —branch of tibial n.
i. Quadratus plantae m.

17. EXTERNAL ANAL SPHINCTER: S3, S4—pudendal n.

## SUMMARY OF MUSCLE INNERVATION

### LOWER EXTREMITY

1. Flexion of hip, sitting up, and adduction of femur mediated by L2, L3, and L4.

2. Extension of knee mediated by L3 and L4 (exception—tensor fasciae latae—L4 to S1).

3. Therefore—dissociation in strength between flexion of the hip and adduction of the thigh on the one hand and extension of the knee on the other points to an exquisite lesion of L2 or L4 (sartorius muscle will be weak if such is the case).

4. Abduction and medial rotation of femur, dorsiflexion of foot, extension of toes, inversion and eversion of foot are all innervated by L4, L5, and S1.

5. If patient can adduct (L2, L3, and L4) the femur and has poor abduction of the femur—a lesion of L5 and S1 is indicated.

6. Poor abduction of femur associated with normal strength in the gastrocnemius, soleus, and muscles of lateral half of foot isolates the lesion to L5.

7. Atrophy of muscles on the lateral half of the sole of the foot with some atrophy and weakness of the calf muscles (gastrocnemius and soleus muscle) and good flexion of *all* the toes—the lesion may be postulated to involve S1 and S2 with sparing of L5.

8. Ability to walk on heels reflects integrity of L4, L5, and S1.

9. Ability to walk on toes reflects integrity of L5, S1, and S2.

10. Injury to common peroneal nerve (especially over head of fibula) results in loss of dorsiflexion and loss of ability to evert the foot—foot is inverted with plantar flexion.

11. Injury to the deep peroneal nerve produces weakness or paralysis of dorsiflexion of foot with ability to evert the foot intact.

12. Injury to superficial peroneal nerve leaves dorsiflexion of foot intact and produces weakness or paralysis of eversion of the foot.

Generally: The anterior thigh muscles represent the upper lumbar cord segments and nerves; anterolateral aspect of the lower leg, the lower lumbar cord segments; the posterior thigh and leg, the lower lumbar and upper sacral cord segments; and the sole, the upper sacral cord segments. The external anal sphincter tone is supplied by the third and fourth sacral cord segments.

# INDEX